Curves®
Member Guide

Written by
Health and Nutrition Counselor
Gary Heavin

Founder & C.E.O., Curves International, Inc.
The World's Largest Fitness Center Franchise

Scripture taken from the Holy Bible, New International Version. Copyright© 1973, 1978, 1984 International Bible Society. Used by permission of Zondervan Bible Publishers.

Nutritional information taken from The Complete Book of Food Counts by Corinne T. Netzer, Copyright© 2000. Published by Dell Publishing a division Random House, Inc., 1540 Broadway, New York, New York 10036. Some nutritional values may be provided by food manufacturers. Unless noted, analysis is given for a single serving. Optional ingredients, ingredients used to garnish and ingredients added "to taste" are not included in the analysis. If an ingredient is listed with an alternative, the figures are calculated for the first choice only.

Manufactured in the United States of America.

Fourth Printing -- September, 2003

Book Design by: Janet Bergin, Mean Mommy Publishing (719-275-6673)
Recipe Development and Editing by: Cathy Bergin, Mean Mommy Publishing (719-275-6673)

~
CONTENTS
~

CURVES MEMBER GUIDE 4
    Chapter I: The Curves Story
    Chapter II: The Curves Difference
    Chapter III: The Curves Workout
    Chapter IV: The Curves Weight Loss Plan
    Chapter V: The Curves Approach to Wellness
              & Nutritional Supplements

RESOURCES 24

PHASE I 77

PHASE II
    Week 1 95
    Week 2 113
    Week 3 131
    Week 4 149
    Week 5 167

PHASE III 185

INDEX 191

He who enjoys good health is rich,
though he knows it not.
—Italian Proverb

CHAPTER I

THE CURVES STORY

As the founder and C.E.O. of the world's largest fitness center franchise, Curves International, Inc., it is my privilege to share the most innovative discoveries in exercise and weight control. Over twenty-eight years ago, I opened my first women's fitness facility and began to coach and guide women through the process of attaining optimal health and weight.

Through the years I developed or made available the most effective methods of health and weight management. They include:

- A strength-training program for women
- A thirty-minute complete workout that fits into busy schedules
- Quality fitness centers designed for women
- Exercise and nutritional guidance at the same location
- A temporary dieting method that produces permanent results
- A business model which is predicated on service
- A community of women who support each other

I wish I could say that I figured it all out easily and recently. When I was a premed major in college, I was learning about physiology at the cellular level. I was not exposed to the standard nutritional theories; instead I studied how the human body actually functions. In other words, I learned how to learn about exercise and weight loss, but I had no bias. I was free to seek the truth.

I was twenty years old and I had been working to put myself through college, but it was becoming apparent that I couldn't afford medical school. Then an opportunity arose to take over a fitness center in Houston, Texas. The facility was about to go out of business when I stepped in. I knew nothing about running a fitness center but I knew about caring for people. I realized that this was an opportunity to treat people before they became ill. I began to take responsibility for the results that the members expected. As their personal trainer, I taught them the proper way to lift weights and perform cardio training. I would weigh and measure them monthly, have them keep food diaries and advise them on their diet. I began to hold weight-loss seminars and offer six-week challenges to the members. At weekly meetings, I monitored calorie intake and results, and discussed willpower and offered support.

I was successful enough to acquire a second location under a management agreement in just over a year. Within a few years, I owned six "women only" fitness centers. I was soon counseling hundreds of women through weekly weight-loss seminars. By the time I was thirty I owned fourteen centers with fifty thousand members. I had written *The Sweet Joy of Sugar Free Living* which utilized the higher-protein, lower-carbohydrate approach to dieting and the Heavin formula for metabolic change.

In my early thirties, I suffered financially through the learning process of experience. However, I retained the information of many years of coaching and counseling and believed that I could create the most effective health and weight-loss program for women.

My wife Diane and I opened the first Curves in Harlingen, Texas, in August of 1992. We were immediately successful but patiently waited two years before opening the second location.

With hundreds of women acquiring the habit of exercise and successfully losing weight, we realized that we should share this program. Franchising seemed to be the perfect vehicle because it worked best when provided by a hometown person who had a passion for serving others. In October of 1995, we opened the first Curves franchise in Paris, Texas. Within ninety days we sold ten franchises. By the end of the first year we had fifty locations. At the end of the second year, we had two hundred and fifty locations and by the end of the third year over six hundred. Today we have over six thousand franchises in the fifty states and nine other countries.

Curves has received many accolades over the last few years. Entrepreneur Magazine has chosen Curves for the following awards:

- "Number 1 Best New Franchise" (two years in a row)
- "Number 2 Best Franchise Overall"
- "The World's Fastest Growing Franchise"
- "Best In Category"

After just seven years in business, we now have one Curves for every two McDonald's restaurants in America. This is a testament to the effectiveness of our program. We knew that the need existed and that we could fill the void in women's fitness.

I recently took the time to finish my formal degree in Health & Nutrition Counseling. Curves is currently underwriting research at Baylor University in an effort to scientifically validate our theories in a laboratory environment. Almost two million women are now using our methods to free themselves from the oppression of obesity and the suffering of chronic disease. The secret of our success is simple. Thirty-minute fitness is something that women will make the time to do. A complete workout, especially one that includes strength training, provides lasting improvement. A convenient and comfortable environment is motivating. Quality nutritional guidance in the same place that you exercise is efficient. A temporary method of dieting with a method to raise metabolism will produce permanent results without permanent dieting.

The Curves community will provide the support and encouragement that will help you succeed with your fitness and weight loss goals. You will find that you can become stronger and healthier in thirty minutes and that you can borrow willpower from a friend.

There's another aspect that has ensured Curves' success. This company has been built on the solid biblical principles of integrity, unity and service. God's will is sought in our business decisions, and then we do our best to carry it out. This commitment includes treating people honestly and fairly and has allowed us to build relationships rather than to just sell franchises or memberships. The astounding growth of this company is His signature. He has provided the opportunity to serve. Our franchisees come from many faiths but all are held to a common value system. It is best expressed in our mission statement.

"We commit our methods and motivation to help people to help themselves in their quest to attain a better quality of life."

If you have any health concerns, you should consult a physician before beginning this or any other fitness and weight-loss program.

CHAPTER II
THE CURVES DIFFERENCE

"Insanity is doing the same thing over and over again and expecting different results."

Albert Einstein

It is reported that 70% of women in America do not exercise on a regular basis. 64% of American adults are overweight and half of those are obese. Type II diabetes is the seventh leading cause of death in America today. Why in a society like ours, are we suffering so? It certainly isn't for lack of information. Is it reasonable to blame ourselves? Are we just too lazy to exercise or too weak to eat less? Perhaps the information is flawed. Would you consider a new approach to exercise, diet and wellness?

Embracing Change
Scott Peck wrote that people change for one of three reasons. To paraphrase: they hit rock bottom. they are desperate, or they learn they can change.

It is very likely that you began past exercise and weight loss program out of emotional reasons such as hitting rock bottom or desperation. These emotional foundations provide poor support for long-term success. As you achieved small successes, you moved from rock bottom or you felt less desperate and your motivation diminished.

With the Curves Program you will learn that you can change. You can become a person who exercises and loses weight successfully. You can begin a program that is reasonable and offers a long-term plan you can believe in.

Curves Community

One of the keys to acquiring a new habit is to create an environment of support. Each Curves location provides just that. You are going to surround yourself with women who share the same goals. As you see others acquiring the habit of exercise and successfully losing weight, you too will find success. Helpful Curves instructors will be there to motivate, train and teach you how to exercise and diet effectively and efficiently. They will be there to hold your hand and to hold you accountable to your exercise and weight loss goals.

Designed for Success

Before Curves, women were second-class citizens in the gyms of America. The equipment was usually made to fit men and the coed environment was uncomfortable for most women. Think of the commercials for other fitness programs; if you didn't look good in a bikini, you probably didn't like their commercials or their facilities. Curves was designed for women and their specific needs. Everything from the comfortable environment to the design of the equipment was intended to provide the best workout a woman could have. As a result, Curves is now the largest fitness franchise in the world and you now have a place where you can acquire the habit of exercise.

The Past Need Not Predict the Future

If you have failed in the past with your exercise and weight loss plans, let's assess your experiences. If your exercise program omitted strength training, you may not have been protecting muscle tissue as you lost weight. With up to 40% of your weight loss in the form of muscle, you drastically lowered your metabolism, thus setting your self up for failure. If you had no exercise regimen while you were dieting, you never experienced the physiological advantages of exercise. Exercise requires energy. Sustained cardiovascular exercise burns more stored fat. The more regularly you exercise, the better your body becomes at accessing fat stores for energy. A complete exercise program will burn more fat and protect metabolically active muscle tissue. Every study shows that those who add exercise to their weight loss program are the most successful.

Low Calorie/Low Fat Dieting

If you followed a traditional low calorie/low fat diet plan, chances are that you were feeding fat while starving muscle. When you consume as little as 1200 calories and only 10 to 15 percent of those calories are in the form of protein, your muscles do not have an adequate supply of essential amino acids. With 65% of your calories coming from carbohydrates, insulin levels are kept high, which feeds and protects fat stores.

Perpetual Dieting

Conventional dieting methods have no way to deal with metabolism which has slowed in response to dieting. Whenever you start to burn stored energy, your body protects itself by becoming more efficient. This survival mechanism lowers metabolism when you are dieting. This is why you hit a plateau. Conventional weight loss programs deal with lower metabolism by requiring a perpetual diet. They may be called maintenance diets or behavior modification, but they are perpetual diets which perpetually lower metabolism and condemn you to a lifetime of dieting and restricted food.

Permanent Results Without Permanent Dieting

With our unique method of raising metabolism following a period of dieting, you will be free from a lifetime of dieting. You will become the master of your weight rather than its slave.

Summary
- Strength training protects and prioritizes muscle tissue and increases the body's energy requirements.
- Exercising while dieting conditions the body to access and burn stored fat.
- Perpetual dieting lowers our metabolism and past dieting methods required that we diet forever to maintain our weight loss because we did not have a method to raise metabolism without regaining our weight.
- A new plan for exercise and weight loss will provide new hope for success.

CHAPTER III

THE CURVES WORKOUT

Thirty-minute Fitness

A common complaint of women is that they just don't have time to exercise. The Curves thirty minute complete workout provides the solution. Our hydraulic resistance strength training machines allow you to perform cardiovascular and strength training at the same time. For thirty minutes, you move around the circuit, changing stations every thirty seconds. You need not rush to a class or worry about a schedule. When you show up, your workout begins. Just jump in anywhere there is a station open and move at the same time and in the same direction as everyone else.

Total Fitness

A complete workout must include warm up, cardio, strength training, cool down and stretching. As you begin the circuit, exercise slowly at each station for the first three to five minutes. As you end the circuit, do the same. This allows your body to warm up and to cool down as you begin and end the workout.

After you warm up you will begin to work harder on each machine. The intensity of a double-positive strength-training machine easily elevates and sustains your target heart rate. As you go around the circuit, you will move from an upper body strength machine to a recovery station to a lower body strength machine and so on. Strength training and cardio are performed simultaneously.

Hydraulic Resistance

The unique features of hydraulic resistance make it possible to perform strength training and cardio at the same time. You will push forward with one muscle group and pull back with the opposing muscles. Gravity does not help or hinder the work. This intensity easily elevates and sustains your target heart rate. By working muscle groups that oppose each other you also work muscles symmetrically or in balance. Two of our machines work in only one direction to effectively target the larger muscle groups.

Safe and Effective

With hydraulic resistance exercise you are moving fluid. This is similar to aquatic exercise, and is inherently safe even for fragile people. There are no weight stacks to manage or decisions to be made. In conventional gyms up to 85% of injuries occur during the eccentric contraction (the lowering of the weight). With a double-positive workout you never lower the weight. You push and pull. The Curves workout provides a strength-training program that many grandmothers and great grandmothers can safely do. Yet it provides resistance and intensity levels that will challenge athletes.

Cardiovascular Training

Cardiovascular training is accomplished by working hard enough to elevate the heart rate to a training (target) level. The heart is a muscle and must perform work to get strong and stay strong. The strength training machines provide the work that elevates the heart to its target level. Every eight minutes you will hear a cue that reminds you to take a ten second heart rate check. Look for the posted heart rate chart and find your age in the column on the left and move across to find your target heart rate. The first column (red - 50%) is the column for people with special health concerns such as high blood pressure, asthma, pregnancy, etc. The second column (yellow - 60%) is where most people should be. The next columns are for those who are more physically fit or athletic. Working out at your target heart rate ensures that you are getting a cardiovascular benefit at a safe yet effective level. It is not necessary to increase your target heart rate percentage as you get in shape. As your physical conditioning improves, you will have to work harder to raise your heart rate to its target level.

Burn Body Fat

Sustained target heart rate activity conditions your body to access stored fat for energy. During the first few minutes of exercise, your muscles will burn energy in the bloodstream and glycogen stored in the muscles. As you continue to exercise, your body will begin to access fat stores for energy. Sustained exercise will continue to burn more fat, and your body will become more proficient at accessing body fat as you exercise on a regular basis.

Optimal Intervals

The thirty-second intervals were chosen because they are the optimal time for a strength training set. Your muscles can "sprint" for about thirty seconds before they begin to exhaust. After an upper body strength machine, you will move to a recovery station for thirty seconds, then to a machine that works the lower body and then to another recovery station. A minute and a half later you will be working an upper body muscle group again. This is the amount of time that a muscle group needs to recover and be ready to sprint again. By alternating muscle groups in this way, you are able to perform cardio and strength training at the same time.

Strength Training

Strength training has long been the missing link in women's fitness. Holding a one-pound dumbbell during an aerobics class was once considered to be strength training. True strength training requires that you move a resistance that is greater than the muscle is accustomed to. Progressive resistance stimulates the muscle to stay strong and firm. Increasing the speed of movement on our machines provides this progressive resistance. The faster you go, the harder it is, because you are moving more fluid through a restricted orifice in the cylinders. You should move the resistance as fast as you are able. This assures that you are "overloading" muscles and achieving the benefits of strength training.

The Intensity Should Be On The Machines

You must work the machines with intensity. Remember that the speed of movement determines the amount of resistance. Strength training achievement requires that you move resistance which is 60 to 80% of your maximum lifting ability. Moving more slowly on the machines means you move less resistance and you may not achieve the full benefits of strength training.

Hesitation Method to Lower Heart Rate

If you find that thirty seconds of working hard on the machines elevates your heart above your training level, you should hesitate at each machine to lower your heart rate to an appropriate level. Simply sit on each machine and wait for five seconds before you begin to work. Five seconds is about 16% of the thirty seconds, which means that you will reduce the amount of work being performed by that percentage. If five seconds does not bring your heart rate down, enough, hesitate for ten seconds. Hesitating, rather than slowing down, on the machines ensures the resistance necessary for strength training while keeping your heart rate at safe training levels.

Benefits of Strength Training

Strong muscles provide the support for joints and vertebrae that keep your body stable and working properly, and bone density increases as a result of load bearing activities. If you are strength training as you lose weight, your body prioritizes muscle tissue and burns more body fat. By protecting muscle mass as you lose weight, you are more likely to reach your weight loss goals and to maintain them.

Rules of Resistance Training

Have your Curves instructor teach you these rules:
- Move across the midline of the muscles
- Keep elbows and knees within the plane of motion
- Move the full range of motion (don't blast your joints)
- Go fast enough to get adequate resistance
- Keep it simple

You Won't Look Like Arnold

Don't worry about gaining too much muscle. You have a preset genetic potential to have a certain amount of muscularity. If you are new to strength training, you may gain 3 to 5 pounds of muscle rather quickly, but it will slow down once you reach your potential for muscle gain. If your body fat percentage is high, you have fat striated throughout the muscles (much like chuck steak). As you burn body fat, you will find that your muscles look smaller.

Exercising Every Day

We recommend that you utilize the Curves workout three times per week due to the need for muscle recovery from strength training. If you desire to work out every day, modify your workout every other day by moving the machines more slowly. By working on the machines more slowly, you will be moving a resistance that is less than 50% of your maximum lifting ability. This should still elevate your heart rate to its target level and provide a cardiovascular workout, but be below the threshold for strength training.

Recovery Stations

We recommend that you "move lively" on the recovery stations, but that means different things for different people. If you are in poor shape or your joints are fragile, you should simply walk in place. If you are in great shape, you may run, do jumping jacks or even the Macarena. Be sure to stay on the board and not step on and off. Keep your movements under control. The level of intensity on the recovery station will not affect your heart rate a great deal. Lowering your heart rate back to your target level will be done on the machines. Do not use dumbbells at the recovery stations. If you feel that you need them, you are holding back on the machines where the real work is performed.

Stretching

Always end your workout with stretching. Your instructor will teach you how to follow the Curves stretching poster. It takes about three minutes to move through all of the stretches. You perform a static stretch by isolating the muscles around a specific joint and extending those muscles completely. Hold the stretch for seven seconds and then extend the muscles further. Being careful not to bob, bounce or pull the muscles, hold each stretch for a total of fifteen seconds. A static stretch is the safest way to stretch and is done at the end of the workout when the muscles are warm. Stretching is important because it helps to maintain range of motion and the integrity of the joints. Be sure to take time at the end of each workout to perform this fifth component of a complete workout.

Core Exercise Program

The Curves workout provides the key components for optimum health: cardiovascular training, strength training and stretching. With hydraulic resistance, the machines will provide greater resistance as you become stronger and more fit. This means that the circuit will continue to provide the work necessary to elevate heart rate and overload muscles. You will never outgrow the intensity of the Curves workout. This thirty minute complete workout may be viewed as a "core workout" that provides an efficient foundation so that you may enjoy a healthy lifestyle. It will enable you to take the stairs, walk your errands, and run and play with your kids and grandkids.

CHAPTER IV

THE CURVES WEIGHT LOSS PLAN

Many of our members who have less than 20 pounds to lose may reach their weight loss goals without having to diet. For women who were not exercising prior to joining Curves, exercise may be such a radical change that the pounds will fall off. When sugar addicts quit eating sugar, the weight often falls off. For those who need an effective weight loss method, we believe we have the best.

The Curves weight loss method is unique in several ways. Our exercise plan includes the cardiovascular component of fitness that conditions the body to better access and burn body fat. The strength-training component prioritizes and protects metabolically active muscle tissue which helps keep metabolism high for more effective loss of body fat and lasting results.

Our diet is unique in that we approach dieting as a temporary condition. It is a time to go from being a food-burning machine to a fat-burning one. This temporary approach to dieting allows us to focus on weight loss, rather than attempting to accomplish every nutritional goal all at the same time. We are able to focus temporarily on weight reduction efforts because we have a method to raise metabolism following a diet. Our metabolic tune-up will increase your metabolism following a diet so that you will not have to diet forever to maintain results.

Both versions of the Curves diet allow for adequate intake of protein which feeds and protects muscle. Both versions limit carbohydrates, which allows you to better access fat stores for energy.

We also provide a test to determine if you are a candidate for the advantages of a high protein/low carbohydrate diet. There are many people who have abused sugar and high carbohydrate processed foods for so long that they have become desensitized to insulin. These people often find that they can eat unlimited amounts of protein, while strictly limiting carbohydrates, and still lose weight. The advantage here is that you don't have to be hungry to lose weight.

We recommend that you not start a diet until after your first month with Curves. If you kick the sugar habit and work out regularly during the first month, you may find that your results are excellent. Don't start dieting until or if it becomes necessary. Remember that the scale measures body fat, muscle, water and clothing, and is not necessarily an accurate measure of your results. Pay attention to the way your clothes feel and the comments that people make. Your instructor will measure your inches and body fat monthly. You will likely gain muscle during your first few months and the scale may not move as much as you hoped. Consider the complete picture, including your energy level, before you choose to diet.

When it's time to diet, ask a Curves instructor to work with you and help you to set goals and determine the best version of our diet for you. You should plan to meet with your instructor on a weekly basis during the six-week weight loss plan while using this book to guide you through Phases I, II and III.

Protein, Fat and Carbohydrates

Foods that are primarily protein include meats, cheeses, eggs, seafood and poultry. Vegetable sources of protein include beans, rice and corn (some foods contain all 3 of the major nutrients). Protein is made up of amino acids that the body uses for energy and to sustain lean tissue and build enzymes, hormones, etc. If a diet is deficient in quality protein the body will give up its protein stores (muscle).

Fats come from animal and vegetable sources. The body uses fat for energy and for maintenance of certain tissues and body processes.

Carbohydrates are sugars that come from fruit (fructose), starches, milk (lactose) and refined sugar (sucrose). Carbohydrates become glucose (sugar) in the bloodstream and are used for energy. Refined carbohydrates such as white flour, (pasta, bagels and most breads), white rice, and sucrose, along with white potatoes, raise blood sugar levels quickly. The body responds by producing insulin. Insulin lowers blood sugar levels by removing glucose from the blood. A small amount of the excess glucose is stored in the muscles and liver as glycogen but the major storage is in the fat cells therefore insulin is considered the fat storage hormone. Carbohydrate addicts often lose their sensitivity to insulin due to years of high insulin levels.

Metabolic rate is the amount of energy your body burns on a given day, measured in calories. The cells of your body require energy, with fat cells requiring small amounts of energy and muscle cells requiring large amounts. A pound of muscle burns up to 50 calories per day at rest. Your body burns fuel from the food you eat or takes it from energy that has been stored as glycogen in the muscles and liver or from fat in the fat cells. A low protein diet combined with exercise that does not include strength training will cause the body to burn lean tissue.

An active person, who also strength trains, will maintain muscle and have a higher metabolic rate. This person can eat more while maintaining a healthy weight. An inactive person who follows a low calorie/low fat/low protein diet has a lower metabolic rate and must eat less to maintain a healthy weight.

Digestion is a high-energy activity. So eating 5 or 6 small meals per day will burn more calories.

Increase Metabolism by Eating

The Journal of the American Medical Association noted in March of 1995, **"Metabolism increases as people eat more and decreases as people eat less."** Do you know anyone who can eat anything they want and never gain weight? As we eat more our bodies increase metabolic rate to prevent us from becoming morbidly obese. We increase metabolism by eating.

Decrease Metabolism by Dieting

Our bodies react to dieting by becoming more efficient. This also is a survival mechanism. As we begin to lose weight on a diet, our bodies sense that we are starving and begin to produce starvation hormones which make us more fuel-efficient. The longer we diet, the heavier the saturation of starvation hormones becomes and the slower our metabolic rate becomes. This explains why weight loss often plateaus and why we must diet forever to maintain weight lost on conventional dieting plans.

However, eating stops the production of starvation hormones and increases metabolic rate. The Cedars-Sinai Hospital Study discovered, **"The human body responds to a fast within about 72 hours."**

The key to raising metabolic rate is to never regain more weight than you can lose within 2 or 3 days. That's how long it takes your body to begin producing starvation hormones. Eating and time will allow starvation hormones to dissipate and will increase metabolism. Perpetual dieting (maintenance diet, behavior modification, etc.) will perpetuate a low metabolism and condemn you to dieting forever.

Phase I

You should begin with Phase I which usually produces quick weight loss and teaches you how to lose weight when you need to. You will use this ability as a tool to help you maintain permanent results without permanent dieting during Phase III. There are two versions of the Curves diet, and you must take the tests to determine which diet will be most effective for you.

HIGHER PROTEIN/LOW CARBOHYDRATE VERSION
Proteins-Eat unlimited quantities of
lean meats, cheeses, eggs, seafood and poultry
Fats-Eat moderate amounts
Carbohydrates-Eat no more than **20** grams per day

LOW CALORIE VERSION
1200 Calories per day - 40% in the form of protein
No more than **60** grams of carbohydrates per day

With both plans, you can enjoy one Curves shake per day and unlimited amounts of free foods. Free foods are vegetables that are low in calories and carbohydrates and contain primarily indigestible roughage, such as lettuces, cabbage, spinach, cauliflower, broccoli, etc.

Be sure to drink 8 glasses of water per day and to take a good multi-vitamin and mineral supplement.

If you have 20 pounds or more to lose, stay on Phase 1 for 2 weeks. If you have 20 pounds or less to lose, move to Phase II after 1 week.

Phase II

HIGHER PROTEIN/LOW CARBOHYDRATE VERSION
Proteins-Eat unlimited quantities of
lean meats, cheeses, eggs, seafood and poultry
Fats-Eat moderate amounts of fats
Carbohydrates-Eat no more than **60** grams per day

LOW CALORIE VERSION
1600 calories per day - 40% in the form of protein
No more than **60** grams of carbohydrates per day

With both plans, you can enjoy one Curves shake per day and unlimited amounts of free foods.

Be sure to drink 8 glasses of water per day and to take a good multi-vitamin and mineral supplement.

Stay on Phase II until:
- You reach your goal
- You hit a plateau
- You need a break from dieting

Phase III

Phase III is not really a diet. It is mostly eating. The objective is to raise metabolism back to pre-diet levels without regaining the weight you lost. The first few pounds that you lose when you diet are water weight. Your body dehydrates as it accesses stored energy and it rehydrates when you begin to eat again.

Establish a low weight and a high weight that allows for a water weight fluctuation and a small amount of body fat. If you want to raise your metabolism up to 2500 calories, you should begin to eat 2500 calories each day. After dieting for weeks, your daily metabolic rate may be as low as 1600 calories. You should expect to gain weight when you eat 2500 calories per day. Remember, eating stops the production of starvation hormones and raises metabolism. The key is to not gain more weight than you can lose in 2 or 3 days, which is the amount of time you can diet before your body responds and begins to produce starvation hormones.

The following example shows the rise of metabolic rate. At 127 pounds. (the low weight), you should begin to eat normally and healthfully. When the scale reaches 130, (the high weight), you will go on the strict Phase I plan for 2 or 3 days. You should find yourself back at 127 and then you begin to eat normally again.

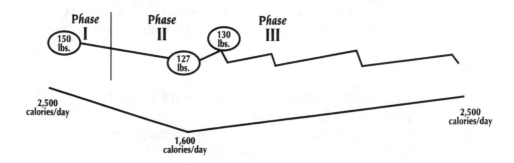

As your body rids itself of starvation hormones, your metabolic rate will increase. You will find that it takes longer and longer to reach your high weight. This indicates that your metabolic rate is increasing. Most people can significantly raise their metabolic rate within a month or two by eating normally and healthfully.

If you have a large amount of weight to lose, you may have to cycle through the 3 phases several times. You should never spend more than a week or two on a frustrating plateau. Phase III will raise your metabolic rate so that you can either continue to lose until you reach your goal or you can maintain your results without having to diet forever.

Two Days Per Month

Except for the extremes of pregnancy, most women gain weight slowly. A half-pound a month becomes 6 pounds a year or 30 pounds in 5 years. Once you have reached your goal and increased your metabolic rate back to pre-diet levels you may find that you can eat normally for as many as 29 days per month. Dieting just 2 or so days per month will burn off the small accumulation that got you into trouble in the past.

CHAPTER V

THE CURVES APPROACH TO WELLNESS & NUTRITIONAL SUPPLEMENTS

"Use it or lose it." When it comes to good health, that's a pretty accurate statement. The human body was made to run, play, work, and to repair itself. It's an amazing machine in that the more you use it, the better its condition. You have begun to use your body in a manner that will keep it working well as long as it has the nutritional building blocks necessary to fuel, protect and repair itself.

We are experiencing an epidemic of chronic disease in America. Type II diabetes has gone from number 100 on the list of common diseases of the last century to the 7th leading cause of death today. Arthritis is prevalent and joint replacements are common for fifty-year olds. Heart disease is the leading cause of death for both men and women, and cancer still stalks the lives of millions. All of these diseases have this in common: exercise and improved nutrition lower their risk significantly.

The medical model in America is designed to treat illness. But we can do better. We can choose wellness. Simply put:

- Perform a complete workout regularly.
- Eat healthy foods and avoid unhealthy ones.
- Make sure that your body has all the nutrients it needs.
- Don't smoke.
- Get regular medical checkups.

Since you have joined Curves, you should see your doctor for a regular physical examination. A good nutritional start would be to exclude processed flour and sugar from your diet. Eat adequate protein and plenty of fruits, vegetables and fiber. If you need to diet to lose body fat, then follow our temporary method that produces permanent results. Even if you eat well, chances are that you are missing nutrients in your diet. Most women do not eat adequate amounts of calcium, and numerous trace minerals are no longer in the foods we eat. Given enough time, a nutrient deficiency may ultimately manifest itself in disease.

What does the human body need?
- Water
- 10 to 12 amino acids
- 3 fatty acids
- 16 vitamins
- 70+ minerals
- Fiber
- Phytonutrients and antioxidants

We can get most of these nutrients from a healthy, well-balanced diet. Vitamins are available in the foods we eat and minerals come from the soil in which the plants are grown. But there is a good chance that we may be missing many of the essential vitamins and minerals.

NPK Fertilization & Minerals

When farmers grow crops, the plants take minerals from the soil and we ingest these minerals from those plants. After a number of years, the soil may become depleted of many of those minerals. Over fifty years ago, scientists discovered that they could grow large and healthy-looking crops just by replacing three minerals in the soil. Fertilization with nitrogen, phosphorous and potassium enabled farmers to continue to grow crops on the same land year after year. A problem became apparent when pests began to attack those unhealthy, nutrient deficient plants and then the pesticide industry was developed. For many years, we have been consuming these plant foods which do not contain all of the nutrients that our bodies need. These nutritional deficiencies are now showing up in chronic diseases such as arthritis, type II diabetes, osteoporosis and heart disease.

Vitamins

Most vitamins are available in the foods we eat, but fast food and processed food may be deficient in vitamins and minerals. The number one vegetable in America today is the french fry, and hectic schedules may make it difficult for you and your family to eat a well-balanced diet. I am a promoter of eating a well-balanced diet and obtaining nutrients from the foods you eat. But I'm also a realist. You probably are not getting all the nutrients you need from your diet. The only way to be sure that you are not missing these essential vitamins and minerals is to supplement them with quality nutritional products. For a thorough explanation of your nutritional needs, read my book *Curves*, published by Putnam.

At the end of this chapter, I will review the Curves supplements which we have developed to meet the needs of women. Let's begin by covering the chronic diseases that can be avoided, or at least postponed, by quality nutrition and a regular and complete exercise program.

Free Radicals

We live in a toxic environment. Smoke from cigarettes, manufacturing and automobiles, chemicals in the things we eat and drink, and dead over-processed foods all contribute to an overabundance of free radicals. Rust that forms on iron is an example of free radical damage. In the body, cells are damaged due to free radical action. This damage is believed to con-tribute to heart disease, cancer, diabetes, arthritis, blindness and aging. Antioxidants protect cells from free radicals. Vitamins E, C and A, beta-carotene, selenium, and zinc, are nutrients that help to defend against free radicals. Grape seed extract, Coenzyme Q10 and Lycopene (which is found in tomatoes) are powerful antioxidants. If you are serious about avoiding disease, you must stop smoking and you must be sure that you are getting adequate antioxidants in your diet or from supplements.

Since it is difficult to acquire the essential nutrients from diet alone, we developed what we believe is the finest multi-vitamin and mineral supple-ment for women. **Curves Complete** provides the full spectrum of quality nutrients, helping to ensure that your body has what it needs, in the right form and ratio, to maintain nutritional health.

Osteoporosis

Of concern to most women is the condition called osteoporosis or "porous bone." Bone loss begins to occur after the age of thirty in most women. It is hastened with menopause, and many women chose hormone replacement therapy as a result. But there is a better method to treat and prevent osteoporosis. Strength training stimulates the manufacture of bone tissue because placing a load on the long bones of the body encourages a bone-building response. If you have the nutritional building blocks of bone in your diet, you should expect bone density to be enhanced. The first study to actually demonstrate the restoration of lost bone density was performed at the University of California by Strause and Saltman, (Journal of Nutrition,

Nutrients Supplemented	% Gain or Loss in Bone Density
1. Placebo	3.52% Loss
2. 25 mg zinc, 5 mg manganese, 2.5 mg copper	1.89% Loss
3. 1000 mg calcium	1.25% Loss
4. 1000 mg calcium + zinc, manganese & copper	**1.48% Gain**

Note: The calcium was citrate and malate, not carbonate.

1994). In a double blind, placebo controlled, two-year study on fifty-nine postmenopausal women, they found the following:

We were unable to find a product on the market that contained a formula similar to the one used in this study which actually demonstrated bone restoration. So we made one. **Curves Essential** is our calcium supplement that contains the nutrients that produced those amazing results.

Arthritis

There are two major types of arthritis: Osteoarthritis and Rheumatoid arthritis. Although they are different diseases, they have in common the damage caused to the joint cartilage. Strength training will help to provide the support that the joints need to work properly. Stretching will help maintain the range of motion and joint function. Losing weight will reduce the stress on the joints, and proper nutrition will help provide the cartilage with the nutrients it needs for cellular health and antioxidants for protection.

The medical regimen for arthritis includes NSAIDS (non-steroidal anti-inflammatory drugs), corticosteroids, antiviral drugs and joint replacement. For the most part, these treat symptoms rather than the underlying cause. They reduce joint swelling and pain but have side effects that may worsen the condition.

Numerous studies have shown that the substances glucosamine and chondroitin are effective in relieving joint pain and reviving the cartilage that provides the cushioning in the joint. In 1980, a Current Medical Research and Opinion article concluded, "It is suggested that…glucosamine sulphate should be considered for the basic therapy of primary or secondary osteoarthritis, mainly because it restores articular function to a certain extent." Glucosamine and chondroitin are natural substances that work by helping to regenerate joint cartilage and assisting in the water retention properties that the cartilage requires. We were unable to find a reliable source for these substances and chose to make our own.

Unlike NSAIDS and other pharmaceuticals, **Curves Integrated** may take longer to provide relief but it treats the cause rather than the symptoms. You must be patient. It is not uncommon to wait a month or two for the effects to be obvious. Some people who no longer have joint cartilage may not obtain adequate relief and benefit.

Type II Diabetes

This insulin resistant type of diabetes is preventable in most people. After years of carbohydrate addiction and the resulting high levels of insulin, the tissues of the body become desensitized to the effects of insulin. The pancreas is ultimately unable to make adequate quantities of insulin to keep blood sugar levels safe. Then uncontrollable levels of blood sugar damage the cells of the body, particularly the eyes, kidneys, nerves and arteries. The medical model recommends drugs, injected insulin and a high carbohydrate (sugar) diet.

We know weight loss and exercise that includes strength training are effective measures in helping to control blood sugar levels. Supplementing with a quality nutritional product may help the body use insulin more effectively. We recommend that people who are addicted to carbohydrates (including white flour, potatoes and rice) break that addiction. Keeping insulin levels low by not eating these simple sugars will help in reacquiring sensitivity to insulin. If you maintain your sensitivity to insulin you may avoid type II diabetes. If you are pre-diabetic, it is possible to move away from diabetes through proper diet and exercise.

Hypertension

High blood pressure has several different causes. Stress is among the most common. Exercise has been shown to be very effective in alleviating stress and lowering blood pressure. It is certainly the preferred method because there are no negative side effects. In addition to mitigating stress, exercise may result in weight reduction and this helps lower blood pressure. Reducing body fat percentage helps the heart and cardiovascular system perform better. Diets that are high in carbohydrates such as sugar, white flour, potatoes and rice, increase levels of insulin which results in retention of water and increased blood volume and blood pressures. A minority of people are salt sensitive and should be careful with salt as it contributes to increased blood volume.

Heart Disease

Heart disease is the leading cause of death in America. Exercise helps keep the heart muscle strong and healthy. Weight control reduces the stress placed on the heart and cardiovascular system. Proper nutrition provides heart healthy nutrients that protect arteries from the damaging effects of free radicals. Reducing unnecessary saturated fat in the diet may help to lower cholesterol levels, but be careful not to rely on foods that are artificial or high in sugar. The famous Harvard Nurses Study found that the nurses who regularly ate margarine instead of butter had almost a third more heart disease. It is believed that butter, because it is natural, is molecularly stable and causes less damage to the carotid arteries than highly unstable artificially-hydrogenated margarine. I believe that the extreme low-fat recommendations and reliance on refined carbohydrates of the past thirty years have contributed to the epidemic of chronic disease and obesity.

Depression

Duke University recently finished a study that found exercise to be more effective than medication for the long-term treatment of depression. 156 men over the age of fifty, who were diagnosed with depression, were divided into three groups. Group One was given the anti-depressant drug Zoloft. Group Two was given Zoloft and began a modest exercise program. Group Three began just an exercise program. After four months, all three groups experienced improvement in their rates of depression. Six months later, however, the Zoloft-only group had a 38 % relapse rate. The exercise and Zoloft group found that 31% of patients had their depression return. The exercise only group found that only 8% of their patients had their depression return.

Exercise is believed to relieve depression due to several factors. Physical activity produces hormones called endorphins which elevate mood. People get a sense of achievement from exercise. Exercise reduces the physiological effects of stress and raises the bar for stressors in our life, so that we are less vulnerable to stress.

Exercise is a great choice in the treatment of depression. It is inexpensive, the side effects are all good and it seems to work better than medication. Pharmaceutical intervention for severe depression can be a wise choice, but long-term treatment should include exercise and proper nutrition.

THE CURVES SUPPLEMENTS

Curves Complete
This liquid multi-vitamin and mineral supplement was formulated to meet the nutritional needs of women. The benefits of this product include:
- All natural vitamins with no synthetics
- The proper ratio of nutrients (synergy)
- An acidic base to enhance absorption
- Plant sourced trace minerals which are recognizable by the body
- Major minerals chelated for best absorption
- Essential fatty acids
- Liquid form which allows for smaller particle size and greater absorption
- Specific nutrients for a woman's needs

We believe we have created the finest nutritional supplement for women. This product should serve as a nutritional foundation for every woman. Each bottle contains the substances, in their ideal form, that a woman's body needs for optimal health. This product includes a unique acidic base liquid to allow for better absorption of minerals. Trace minerals are in organic form and include minute quantities of essential substances which are rarely found in other products, while major minerals are in chelated form for most efficient absorption. The synergistic ratio of nutrients works together for optimal effectiveness. Be sure to shake it well before using. The dosage is one ounce per 100 pounds of body weight. You can mix it with juice or water. Be sure to take it with meals, and never on an empty stomach.

Curves Integrated

Our joint support formula contains glucosamine and chondroitin sulfates along with MSM and other minerals and vitamins. We believe this product promotes joint health and relieves swelling and pain. Along with an exercise program that includes stretching and strength training, weight reduction, and proper nutrition, we believe that this may be the best overall supplement for treatment and prevention of many types of arthritis.

Curves Essential

Our calcium supplement includes the type of calcium that has been shown to restore bone density in the Strause & Saltman osteoporosis medical study. It also includes other minerals and nutrients that have been demonstrated to be effective in the treatment and prevention of osteoporosis.

Curves Herbal-Fem

Along with **Curves Essential**, this product provides an alternative to hormone replacement therapy. As a woman transitions from her child-bearing years, her body has mechanisms to maintain quality of life. Among these is the ability of the adrenal glands to manufacture hormones that help maintain a woman's biochemistry. If poor nutrition and stress have disabled the adrenal glands, Herbal-Fem helps with nutrients and herbal remedies that have long proven effective in treating the symptoms of menopause.

Curves PMS Formula

This formula utilizes a blend of nutrients and herbal remedies that may help to balance the effects of monthly hormonal fluctuations.

Curves Protein Shake

Our meal replacement shake is a delicious drink that is rich in nutrients, including soy protein with isoflavones, a natural estrogen. Each shake contains over twenty grams of protein and has only twenty grams of carbohydrates. The herbal blend speeds the digestive process and helps to detoxify the body. It comes in chocolate and vanilla flavors and uses no artificial sweeteners or sucrose. When you have to diet, it provides a wonderful reward that will help you to stay motivated. You should mix it up with ice and skim or soy milk, and one per day is considered a free food on our diet.

What Should I Take

Every woman should utilize the solid nutritional foundation of Curves Complete. Our other products are designed to supplement this foundation and should only be taken by those with the specific needs.

Medical Advice

If you are on medications, you should consult with your doctor before taking these or any supplements.

These statements have not been evaluated by the Food and Drug Administration. These products are not intended to diagnose, treat, cure or prevent any disease.

~
RESOURCES
~

Progress Charts .25

Tests 28

Test Results 30

Phase I Explanation 30

Free Foods List .31

Free Foods Salad 32

Helpful Information 34

Curves Shake Variations 43

How to Use the Food Diary Pages 44

Substitutions 46

Personal Food Directory 47

Carbohydrate & Calorie Charts 48

Vitamin & Mineral Charts 56

Recipes 58

Curves Diet Checklist 75

Phase I Shopping List 76

MEASUREMENT CHART

Keeping track of your progress is important.

WEEK 1 - BEGINNING MEASUREMENTS

Bust _____
Waist _____
Abdomen _____
Hip _____
Thigh _____
Calf _____
Arm _____
Weight _____
Body fat % ____
Fat lbs. _____
Date _____

WEEK 4 - MEASUREMENTS

Bust _____
Waist _____
Abdomen _____
Hip _____
Thigh _____
Calf _____
Arm _____
Weight _____
Body fat % ____
Fat lbs. _____
Date _____

WEEK 6 - ENDING MEASUREMENTS

Bust _____
Waist _____
Abdomen _____
Hip _____
Thigh _____
Calf _____
Arm _____
Weight _____
Body fat % ____
Fat lbs. _____
Date _____

GOAL MEASUREMENTS

Bust _____
Waist _____
Abdomen _____
Hip _____
Thigh _____
Calf _____
Arm _____
Weight _____
Body fat % ____
Fat lbs. _____
Date _____

WEIGHT LOSS CHART

Write your beginning weight in the top box in the left column and enter one pound decreases down the column. Place an X in the corresponding weekly weight amounts. Place your goal weight in the goal box. This graph will help you visualize your path to success.

Weight	Beginning	Week 1	Week 2	Week 3	Week 4	Week 5	Ending	Goal
185	X							
184								
183								
182		X						
181								
180			X					
179				X				

Weight	Beginning	Week 1	Week 2	Week 3	Week 4	Week 5	Ending	Goal

EXERCISE CHART

Keep a record of weekly exercise. Each day place an X in the box for each ten minutes of exercise performed. Write the type of exercise and how much energy you felt afterward, on a scale of 1 to 5, with 5 being the highest.

Week #	Day or Date	Minutes per day Each box = 10 minutes								Type of Exercise	Post Exercise Energy Level 1 to 5 (most)

TEST I

SYMPTOMS OF
CARBOHYDRATE INTOLERANCE

(Check any symptoms you experience on a regular basis)

____Nervousness

____Irritability

____Fatigue and exhaustion

____Faintness, dizziness, cold sweats, shakiness, weak spells

____Depression

____Drowsiness, especially after meals or in mid-afternoon

____Headaches

____Digestive disturbances with no apparent cause

____Forgetfulness

____Insomnia

____Needless worry

____Mental confusion

____Rapid pulse, especially after eating certain foods

____Muscle pains

____Antisocial behavior

____Overly emotional crying spells

____Lack of sex drive

____Leg cramps and blurred vision

____Shortness of breath, sighing and excess yawning

____Cravings for starch and sugar-rich foods

____**Total**

TEST II

CARBOHYDRATE INTOLERANCE

(Check all statements that apply to you)

____You are more than 25 pounds overweight

____You have had a tendency to be overweight all of your life

____You have been overweight since you were a child

____You have a poor appetite and often skip meals

____You have food cravings that temporarily go away when starchy or sugary foods are eaten

____There are foods that you feel you absolutely could not do without

____Your waist is bigger than your hips

____You checked most or all of the symptoms on Test 1

____**Total**

~

TEST III

CALORIE SENSITIVITY

(Check all statements that apply to you)

____You had a normal body weight when younger but slowly gained weight after age 30

____You are presently overweight, but by less than 25 pounds

____You have a normal appetite and get hungry at meal times

____You have few, if any, food cravings

____You have maintained the same basic eating habits all of your life

____You eat three meals per day

____You have gained a certain amount of extra body weight but seem to have tapered off (not continued to steadily gain more and more weight)

____You checked few or none of the symptoms on Test 1

____**Total**

TEST RESULTS

If you agreed with more statements on Test II, (the carbohydrate-intolerance quiz), you should be successful on a higher-protein diet. If you agreed with more statements on Test III, (the calorie-sensitive quiz), you should restrict your calorie intake. If you agreed with a similar number on both, you can probably start with a higher protein diet and enjoy its advantages, but you will need to restrict calories later to continue losing weight.

PHASE I

Phase I is the strictest part of the plan. You will choose the most advantageous method of dieting for you, based on the tests on pages 28 and 29. If the tests show that you are carbohydrate intolerant, you may enjoy the advantage of a higher protein and lower carbohydrate plan. The advantage of this plan is that you can eat more food and still lose weight. However, you must limit your carbohydrates to 20 grams per day (not counting free foods).

If the tests show that you are calorie sensitive, you must eat fewer calories, as well as limiting carbohydrates. The calorie sensitive plan calls for 1200 calories and 60 grams of carbohydrates per day (not counting free foods).

If you are one of the 25% who seem to be both carbohydrate and calorie sensitive, you may start with the higher protein plan. If you haven't lost any weight within a few days, go to the calorie restricted plan, or if your weight loss stops following several weeks of success with the higher protein plan, move to the calorie restricted plan.

Stay on the stricter Phase I plan for one or two weeks depending on the amount of weight you need to lose. If you have less than twenty pounds to lose, one week is sufficient. If you have twenty or more pounds to lose, two weeks is appropriate.

It is very motivating to lose weight quickly. However, for periods longer than two weeks, you need wider variety and larger amounts of food than Phase I provides. Phase I will allow you to acquire the skill and confidence to lose weight when you need to. This tool is an important part of Phase III.

Enjoy your free foods and the variety they provide. One Curves shake per day (made with skim milk) will give you a moment of pleasure by providing a treat.

FREE FOODS

You may have as much of these vegetables as you like. The closer to raw that you eat them, the better. Their calorie and carbohydrate content is not counted in your daily totals.

asparagus
bamboo shoots
broccoli
brussels sprouts
cabbage (any kind)
cauliflower
celery
cucumbers
garlic
green leafy vegetables
lettuce (any kind)
mushrooms
onions (non-sweet)
peppers (any kind)
pickles (dill only)
radishes
sauerkraut
snow peas
spinach
sprouts
summer squash
zucchini

~

Curves shake made with
8 ounces of skim milk (one per day)

~

Flavoring choices:
yellow mustard
lemon juice

FREE FOODS SALAD

Any time salad is listed in your meal plan, use as much as you like of the free foods (see page 31 for a list of free foods). Add any of the following items according to your tastes and how many carbohydrates and calories you want to have. Use the blank lines to record your favorite salad additions.

FOOD ITEM	AMOUNT	CARBOHYDRATES	CALORIES
Artichoke hearts, water packed	3 pcs.	3 grams	18
Avocado	1/2	6 grams	162
Blue cheese, crumbled	1 Tbsp.	0 grams	30
Carrots	1/2 cup	6 grams	24
Egg, hard boiled	1	0 grams	75
Olives, black, sliced	1 Tbsp.	1 gram	9
Tomato	1 small	6 grams	30
Soy nuts, honey-roasted	1 Tbsp.	3 grams	29
Sunflower seed kernels	1 Tbsp.	1 gram	47

Don't forget the dressing—use something you like. Remember that fat free dressings often have more carbohydrates than the regular ones. (See page 33 for a Salad Dressing Table)

HINT: Each day's meal plan is deliberately short of calories and carbs so that you have room to add what you like to your salad. Be sure you add enough stuff to make your salads enjoyable.

SALAD DRESSINGS

There is a dizzying array of salad dressings at most super-markets. For Phase I, you need a salad dressing with few carbohydrates and limited calories, but it must taste good enough for you to enjoy it. Can you find a salad dressing with less than 4 carbohydrates and less than 50 calories in a serving of 2 tablespoons?

For Phase II, you can probably have higher calorie and carb salad dressings. You might want to keep several on hand to provide variety.

Record your favorites in the table below.

BRAND	KIND	PER 2 TABLESPOONS	
		CARBOHYDRATES	CALORIES

BASIC KITCHEN TOOLS

kitchen scale
measuring cups
measuring spoons
colander

❧

paring knife
utility knife
vegetable peeler
cutting board
grater

❧

saucepan
sauté pan
skillet
broiler pan
meat thermometer
timer

❧

can opener
mixing bowls
hand mixer
blender
whisk
wooden spoon

MEASUREMENT EQUIVALENTS

dash = less than $1/8$ teaspoon

3 teaspoons = 1 tablespoon

4 tablespoons = $1/4$ cup

$5 1/3$ tablespoons = $1/3$ cup

8 tablespoons = $1/2$ cup

$10 2/3$ tablespoons = $2/3$ cup

12 tablespoons = $3/4$ cup

14 tablespoons = $7/8$ cup

16 tablespoons = 1 cup

8 ounces = 1 cup

1 cup = $1/2$ pint

2 cups = 1 pint

16 ounces = 2 cups

2 pints (4 cups) = 1 quart

4 quarts (liquid) = 1 gallon

8 quarts (solid) = 1 peck

4 pecks = 1 bushel

16 ounces = 1 pound

Curves safety tip:

Ground beef patties and loaves are safe when they reach 160° F in the center; ground poultry patties and loaves are safe at 165° F.

PANTRY ESSENTIALS

chopped garlic (in a jar)
lemon juice
lemon pepper seasoning
light mayonnaise
olive oil
prepared yellow mustard
salad dressing
Curves shake mix

BASIC COOKING TERMS

Bake – To cook covered or uncovered in an oven or oven-type appliance. For meats cooked uncovered, it's called roasting.

Baste – To moisten foods during cooking with pan drippings or special sauce to add flavor and prevent drying.

Beat – To make mixture smooth by adding air with a brisk whipping or stirring motion using spoon, whisk or electric mixer.

Blend – To thoroughly mix two or more ingredients until smooth and uniform.

Boil – To cook in liquid at boiling temperature (212 degrees at sea level) where bubbles rise to the surface and break. For a full rolling boil, bubbles form rapidly throughout mixture.

Braise – To cook slowly with a small amount of liquid in tightly covered pan on top of range or in oven.

Broil – To cook by direct heat, usually under broiler in oven with door partially open or over coals.

Chop – To cut in pieces about the size of peas with knife, chopper or blender.

Cool – To remove from heat and let stand at room temperature.

Cream – To beat with spoon or electric mixer until mixture is soft and smooth. When applied to blending shortening and sugar, mixture is beaten until light and fluffy.

Cut in – To mix shortening with dry ingredients using pastry blender or knives.

Dice – To cut food in small cubes of uniform size and shape.

Glaze – A mixture applied to food which hardens or becomes firm and adds flavor and a glossy appearance.

Grill – An outdoor or indoor cooking method in which food is placed on a metal grid directly over a heat source, whether charcoal, wood, gas or electric coil. It also refers to cooking on a hot, flat metal surface.

Julienne – To cut food into long, thin strips.

Marinate – To allow food to stand in a liquid to tenderize or add flavor.

Mince – To cut or finely chop food into very small pieces.

Poach – To cook in hot liquid, being careful that food holds its shape.

Precook – To cook food partially or completely before final cooking or reheating.

Roast – To cook uncovered without water added, usually in an oven

Sauté – To brown or cook in small amount of butter or oil.

Steam – To cook in steam with or without pressure. A small amount of boiling water is used, and more water being added during steaming process if necessary.

Toss – To mix ingredients lightly.

Truss – To secure fowl or other meat with skewers during cooking.

Whip – To beat rapidly to incorporate air to produce expansion, usually in heavy cream or egg whites.

BASIC SPICES

Beef:
basil
chili powder
cumin
coriander
cilantro
oregano
parsley flakes
rosemary
sage
tarragon

Pork:
basil
chili powder
cumin
coriander
cilantro
oregano
parsley flakes
rosemary
sage

Lamb:
cumin
coriander
cilantro
oregano
rosemary
saffron

Chicken:
basil
chili powder
cumin
coriander
cilantro
ground mustard
oregano
parsley flakes
poultry season-
ing
rosemary
saffron
sage
tarragon

Turkey:
basil
chili powder
cumin
coriander
cilantro
oregano
parsley flakes
rosemary
sage
tarragon

Seafood:
basil
chili powder
cumin
coriander
cilantro
lemon pepper
oregano
rosemary
saffron
sage
tarragon

Shellfish:
basil
chili powder
cumin
coriander
cilantro
lemon pepper
paprika
parsley flakes
rosemary
tarragon

HOW TO COOK MEAT AND FISH

To cook meat and fish without adding fat and calories, grilling and broiling are good choices. Season meat or fish to your taste (be adventurous with spices) and grill or broil to desired doneness. Fish is fully cooked when it becomes opaque and flakes easily. Marinades can contribute delicious flavor while adding minimal carbohydrates and calories. Check them out at your supermarket.

Fish may be baked in the oven at 375°F, but be sure to add some liquid and cover your baking dish. This will keep your fish moist. Good liquids to add are: chicken broth, lemon juice, wine or Italian dressing.

Meats and fish always taste great sautéed. You may use one tablespoon of olive oil or a nonstick spray in the sauté pan. Season meat or fish and cook to the desired doneness.

Chicken, pork and beef can be nicely cooked in a crock pot with some added liquid. The final result will be very tender and flavorful.

Experiment with these cooking methods to find your favorite.

DIETING ON THE GO

If you are working outside your home, this diet presents some challenges. You need to be able to take food with you and eat it at appropriate times.

Use your imagination about switching around the order of your meals. You might want to eat a meal in the morning and make a shake to take and drink later. Many of the meals are very portable and don't even require heating up. If you have access to a microwave oven, you have more options.

You will need a number of small containers and access to either a refrigerator or a small cooler. To take a salad, mix the leafy ingredients in one container and the wet ingredients (such as cucumber, tomato, etc.) in another. You can pack a measured amount of dressing in a very small container.

The key to making this diet work is planning.

FEEDING YOUR FAMILY
WHILE YOU FOLLOW
THE CURVES PLAN

On a daily basis, it is much too complicated to cook different meals for your family and yourself. The Curves Weight Loss Method meals are great for your family dinners. You may want to add a starch to the meal, such as rice, pasta, potatoes, grits or dressing. Another good addition to the meal is fruit. Of course, you need to not eat the starch nor the fruit in order to keep following the diet plan.

If you have trouble finding the will power to resist the foods that are not on your diet plan, it may help to fill the plates in the kitchen so that the serving dishes are not on the table while you eat.

Your family will probably love to have a chance to support your dieting efforts and everyone may gain some good new eating habits.

TIPS FOR EATING OUT

Given the hectic pace of life and our need for convenience, the average American eats away from home in restaurants about 8 times per month. A study at Tufts University in Boston found that the more often people eat out, the fatter they become. Here are a few tips to help you balance the need for convenience and still maintain a healthy diet plan while eating out.

• **Control portion sizes.** Restaurants of all types give you more food than the normal portion to create the appearance of price value. To combat this, share an entree with a friend or box half and take it home for another meal. You don't have to clean your plate to get your money's worth.

• **Drink water with your meal** and cut calories and cost. The average glass of soda or sweetened tea has about 150 calories and 40 carbohydrates.

• **Avoid the "urge to splurge"** each time you eat out. If you only eat out once a month, dessert is a fine part of an overall healthy eating plan. But with most of us eating out twice a week or more, it becomes more important to pass on the high calorie, high fat and high sugar treats each time. If you must have a dessert, order one and share it with others in your party.

• **Get it on the side.** Dressing, gravy, and sauce can add a lot of carbs and calories. Order these on the side to better control the amount you eat.

• **Ask lots of questions** about your selection. How is it cooked? What is served with it? Choose meats that are steamed, grilled, baked or broiled instead of fried. Trim visible fat from meat or skin from poultry.

• **You can't go wrong** with plain grilled meat or fish and salad or free vegetables.

• **Eat slowly and talk more.**

WATER

A woman's body is usually 50-55% water. Body water performs three essential functions:

1. helps give structure and form to the body by plumping up tissues,
2. creates the water-based environment necessary for the chemical actions and reactions that make up the body's metabolism and sustain life,
3. provides the means for maintaining a stable body temperature.
4. protects the kidneys and helps detoxify the body

Obviously, it is very important that we drink adequate water every day. Our health depends on it, and so does our beauty. Drinking plenty of water helps to maintain good skin tone and color. It is also of great assistance in maintaining normal digestion.

We all need to drink at least 8 (8-ounce) glasses of water every day. (2 quarts)

Caffeinated beverages act as a mild diuretic, and so they should not be counted as a part of your daily water intake.

FIBER

Fiber is a very important part of our diet. Eating plenty of fiber can have a positive impact on diabetes, heart disease, colon cancer and other gastrointestinal diseases.

The recommended daily allowance of dietary fiber is 20 to 35 grams per day (for adults). This goal can be easily achieved through generous consumption of whole grains, legumes, vegetables, fruits, seeds and nuts.

The Curves Weight Loss Method may have less fiber than you are accustomed to. If you are troubled by irregularity, cramps or other symptoms, you may want to consider supplementing your fiber intake. Powdered fiber can be added to your daily protein shake (about 1 teaspoon) or to yogurt. Your supermarket or pharmacy probably has a number of fiber supplement options. Finally, be sure to drink plenty of water to ease digestive symptoms.

A great way to increase your total fiber intake is to eat $1/4$ cup of a bran cereal (such as Fiber One) with $1/4$ cup skim milk (no sugar allowed!) Use the table below to record the carb, calorie, and fiber counts of some of the cereals you might try.

	amount	grams of carbohydrate	calories	fiber
skim milk	$1/4$ cup	3	21	0
Fiber One	$1/4$ cup	12	30	6.5
All Bran	$1/4$ cup	12	40	5.5

SEVEN WAYS TO SIZE UP YOUR PORTIONS

1 3 ounces of meat is about the size and thickness of a deck of playing cards or an audiotape cassette.

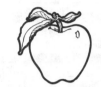 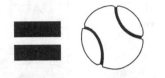

2 A medium apple or peach is about the size of a tennis ball.

 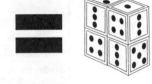

3 1 ounce of cheese is about the size of 4 stacked dice.

 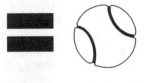

4 ½ cup of ice cream is about the size of a racquetball or tennis ball.

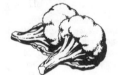 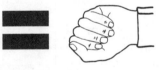

5 1 cup of broccoli or mashed potatoes is about the size of your fist.

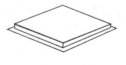 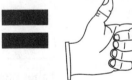

6 1 teaspoon of butter or peanut butter is about the size of the tip of your thumb.

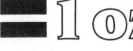

7 1 ounce of nuts or small candies equals one handful.

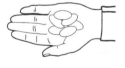  = 1 oz.

HOW TO READ
A NUTRITION LABEL

The nutrition label can be found on food packages in your supermarket. What you see on the label—the nutritional information and ingredient list—is required by the government.

Serving Size: Similar food products now have similar serving sizes. This makes it easier to compare foods.

Calories listed are per individual serving.

Vitamins and minerals: Only two vitamins, A and C, and two minerals, calcium and iron, are required on the food label. A food company can voluntarily list other vitamins and minerals in the food.

Nutrition Facts

Serving Size 1/2 cup (114g)
Servings Per Container about 4

Amount Per Serving

Calories 90   Calories from Fat 30

	% Daily Value
Total Fat 3g	**5%**
Saturated Fat 0g	**0%**
Cholesterol 0mg	**0%**
Sodium 300mg	**13%**
Total Carbohydrate 13g	**4%**
Dietary Fiber 3g	**12%**
Sugars 3g	
Protein 3g	

Vitamin A   80% • Vitamin C   60%
Calcium   4% • Iron   10%

*Percent Daily Values are based on a 2,000 calorie diet. Your daily values may be higher or lower depending on your calorie needs.

	Calories:	2,000	2,500
Total Fat	Less than	65g	80g
Sat Fat	Less than	20g	25g
Cholesterol	Less than	300mg	300mg
Sodium	Less than	2,400mg	2,400mg
Potassium	Less than	3,500mg	3,500mg
Total Carbohydrate		300mg	375g
Dietary fiber		25g	30g

Label numbers: Numbers on the nutrition label may be rounded.

% Daily Value: % Daily Value shows how a food fits into a 2,000 calorie reference diet. You can use % Daily Value to compare foods and see how the amount of nutrients in a serving of food fits in a 2,000 calorie reference diet.

Total grams of **carbohydrates** are per individual serving

Approximate number of calories per gram:

Fat – 9   Carbohydrate – 4   Protein – 4   Alcohol – 7

CURVES SHAKE
VARIATIONS

The prescribed way to make the shake is with 8-ounces of skim milk (and 4 or 5 ice cubes, if you like it frosty and slushy). The Curves Shake comes in chocolate and vanilla flavors. Here are some different ways to make the shake and the changes to your carbohydrate and calorie counts.

Soy milk is a suitable substitute for those that are lactose intolerant.

- Use 8 ounces of 1% milk (tastes a little creamier)
  Add 0 carbohydrates and 30 calories.
- Use 8 ounces of 2% milk (tastes much creamier)
  Add 0 carbohydrates and 40 calories
- Use 8 ounces of whole milk (tastes rich and creamy)
  Add 0 carbohydrates and 70 calories
- Add 1 teaspoon real vanilla extract
  Add 1 carbohydrate and 10 calories
- Add $1/8$ to $1/4$ teaspoon mint extract
  Add 0 carbohydrate and 5 calories
- Add $1/4$ to $1/2$ teaspoon orange extract
  Add 0 carbohydrate and 11 calories
- Add $1/2$ teaspoon pure almond extract
  Add 0 carbohydrates and 11 calories
- Add 1 tablespoon coffee liquor
  Add 8 carbohydrates and 58 calories
- Add 1 tablespoon brandy
  Add 0 carbohydrates and 32 calories
- Instead of ice cubes, add $1/2$ of a frozen banana and whip up in a blender
  Add 13 carbohydrates and 53 calories
- Add any fruit from another meal in the same day

Use your imagination—you'll be surprised at the delicious combinations you can make up.

GUIDE TO FOOD DIARY ICONS

Mark out or fill in each icon
as you complete it.

Water: 🥛 —each glass
represents one
8-ounce glass of
water consumed

Vitamins: ⬭ —each
capsule is a
reminder to take
vitamin supplements

Daily Exercise: ♡ —check
off your workout for
the day: either the
Curves Workout or
something else such
as walking, biking,
pilates, dance,
stretching, etc. Write
down the type of
exercise and how
long you did it.

HOW TO USE THE FOOD DIARY PAGES

Each day of this diet has its own food diary page on which your meals are laid out for you. Feel free to eat the meals in any order that works for you. It is very important to eat all six meals every day, which means that you will be eating every three or four hours. If you make a substitution, cross out what you did not eat and write in what you did eat. Check off the foods you do eat. Be sure to record the carbs and calories for the food you ate. Be sure to record everything you add to your Free Foods Salads, including dressing. Some foods have recipes provided in this book. At the top corner of the recipe page you can find the carb and calories totals to use in your diary. Free foods are not counted in your daily totals.

Record your water consumption by crossing out the water glass icons at the bottom of each food diary. You may want to use the vitamin pill icons to remind yourself to take vitamins and supplements. Record your exercise for the day.

At the end of the day, total up your carbs and calories. A sample completed food diary page can be found on the next page.

One of the most common reasons women are not successful on this diet is that they don't eat enough calories. If you are regularly below 1000 net calories, you must eat more calories without exceeding your carb limit.

Day: Sample Completed Food Diary

			Carbs	Calories
Meal 1	✓	½ cup 1% fat cottage cheese	5	80
		~~½ cup strawberries~~	~~6~~	~~23~~
		¼ cup blueberries	7	27
Meal 2	✓	Curves shake with 8 oz. skim milk	FREE	FREE
Meal 3	✓	4 ounces 93% lean ground beef, broiled	0	160
	✓	Free Foods Salad		
		Salad Dressing (your choice)	2	30
		1 T. blue cheese	0	30
		½ tomato	3	47
Meal 4	✓	⅔ cup tuna salad (recipe page 61)	3	258
	✓	*2 Rye Krisp crackers	11	60
		1 peach	9	37
Meal 5	✓	6 ounces chicken breast, broiled	0	186
	✓	Parmesan Vegetable Stir Fry (recipe page 73)	0	175
Meal 6	✓	2 ounces lean ham	0	67
	✓	*1 small apple	20	80

Water: 🥛🥛🥛🥛🥛🥛🥛🥛

Vitamins: 💊💊💊

Totals for Day	60	1237

Today's Exercise:

Curves Workout ✓

or

Aerobic ♡

_____

_____

Strength Training ♡

_____

_____

Stretching ♡

_____

_____

If you are following the carbohydrate-restricted version, don't eat the foods that are marked with an asterisk (*). You are allowed to eat unlimited quantities of no-carb foods and free foods.

SUBSTITUTIONS

RESOURCES

3 ounces tofu	=	1 egg
	=	3 ounces turkey
	=	3 ounces chicken
strawberries	=	blueberries
	=	raspberries
3 sausage links	=	5 ounces lean ham
4 ounces salmon	=	8 ounces orange roughy
plain lowfat yogurt	=	1% fat cottage cheese
2 Rye Krisp crackers	=	2 Harvest Multigrain crackers
Broccoli	=	Cauliflower
1 ounce Havarti cheese	=	1 ounce Cheddar cheese
1/2 cup cantaloupe	=	1/2 cup watermelon
	=	1/4 cup seedless grapes

Figure out some of your own substitutions.

_____ = _____

_____ = _____

_____ = _____

46

YOUR PERSONAL FOOD DIRECTORY

It has been said that most people eat fewer than 15 foods on a regular basis. One of the keys to good nutrition is variety, so it is important to work at incorporating more and different foods into your regular diet.

A great tool for developing your own personal healthy eating plan is a Personal Food Directory with nutritional information for each food you regularly eat. Most people find it helpful to divide their Directory into types of foods such as: dairy products, fats, fruits, starches, protein, nuts, vegetables, prepared foods and other. Within each type, alphabetizing your list can make looking up the nutritional information more efficient. At a minimum, you will want to list serving size, calories and carbohydrates for each food entry. You may also want to know the protein, fat, fiber, cholesterol and sodium content of the foods.

Your best source of nutritional information is the package the food comes in. If there is no information on the package, you should be able to look the food up in a book such as *The Complete Book of Food Counts*, by Corinne T. Netzer.

There are also some computer programs that can assist you in making your Personal Food Directory.

The next 7 pages (pages 48-54) contain lists of some common foods. Add your favorites at the bottom of each list, or write them on the chart on page 55.

This information is vital to your ability to make good food choices.

VEGETABLES

	amount	grams of carbohydrate	calories
Artichoke hearts, water packed	3 pieces	3	18
*Asparagus, sliced	1/2 cup	4	22
Avocado	1/2 of medium	6	162
*Broccoli florets	1 cup	5	24
*Cabbage, shredded	1 cup	4	16
Carrots, sliced	1 cup	11	48
*Cauliflower florets	1 cup	5	26
*Celery	1/2 stalk	1	3
Corn (baby)	1/4 cup	2	15
Corn (whole kernel)	1/2 cup	13	66
*Cucumber, sliced	1/8 of medium	1	5
*Garlic	1 clove	1	4
Green beans, cut	1/2 cup	4	20
*Green Onion	1 piece	0	1
*Green onion, sliced	1 tablespoon	1	4
*Lettuce leaves	4 large	3	12
*Lettuce leaves, torn up	2 cups	4	16
*Mushrooms, sliced	1/2 cup	4	21
Olives, ripe, sliced	1/2 cup	1	9
*Onion	1/2 of medium	14	60
*Onion, chopped	1 cup	14	60
Peas, green	1/2 cup	11	60
*Pepper, green & red bell	1 medium	5	20
*Pickles, dill	1 medium	3	12
Pickles, sweet	1 medium	10	41
*Radishes	1 piece	0	1
*Sauerkraut	1/2 cup	5	20
*Snow peas	1/2 cup	7	30
*Spinach, fresh	1 cup (packed)	2	12
*Summer Squash, sliced	1/2 cup	3	13
Tomato	1/2 of medium	3	15
Tomato paste	1 tablespoon	3	12
V-8 juice	1 cup (8 ounce)	10	46
*Zucchini, sliced	1/2 cup	2	9

*Free Foods

FRUITS

	amount	grams of carbohydrate	calories
Apple, with peel	1 small	20	80
Banana	1/2 of medium	13	53
Blueberries	1/4 cup	7	27
Cantaloupe, cubed	1/2 cup	6	25
Cranberries, dried & sweetened	1/3 cup	33	130
Grapefruit	1/2 of medium	12	46
Grapes, seedless	1/2 cup	14	57
Lime juice	1 1/2 tablespoons	1	5
Nectarine	1 medium	16	67
Orange	1 medium	16	65
Orange juice	2 1/2 tablespoons	4	17
Orange juice, from concentrate	1 cup (8 ounce)	28	110
Peach, peeled	1 medium	9	37
Plum	1 medium	9	36
Raspberries	1/4 cup	4	17
Strawberries	1/2 cup	6	23
Watermelon, cubed	1/2 cup	6	25

PROTEIN

	grams of carbohydrate	calories
Poultry		
4 oz. chicken breast, grilled or broiled	0	124
4 oz. fajita chicken	0	120
4 oz. turkey breast, grilled or broiled	0	120
4 oz. deli turkey breast	4	120
Beef		
4 oz. broiled sirloin	0	215
4 oz. roast beef, deli	4	120
1/4 lb. hamburger patty (93% lean)	0	160
1/4 lb. hamburger patty (96% lean)	0	130
Pork		
4 oz. center cut pork chop, lean, broiled	0	150
4 oz. pork loin	0	150
3 oz. lean ham	0	100
4 oz. light smoked sausage	8	220
Fish		
6 oz. tuna, packed in water	0	180
4 oz. salmon, broiled	0	207
4 oz. rainbow trout	0	200
1/4 lb. shrimp, broiled or grilled	0	120
8 oz. orange roughy	0	216
Eggs		
large	trace	75
Tofu		
3 oz. tofu (extra firm)	1	90

NUTS

	amount	grams of carbohydrate	calories
Almonds, roasted & salted	1 ounce	4	180
Cashews, roasted & salted	1 ounce	7	170
Macadamia nuts, roasted & salted	1 ounce	3	220
Peanuts, dry roasted	1 ounce	5	160
Peanut Butter	2 tablespoons	7	190
Pistachio nuts, in shells	2 ounces	7	170
Soy nuts, honey roasted	2 tablespoons	5	58
Sunflower seed kernels, roasted & salted	1 tablespoon	1	47

FATS

	amount	grams of carbohydrate	calories
Butter	1 tablespoon	0	102
Mayonnaise	1 tablespoon	0	100
Mayonnaise, light	1 tablespoon	1	50
Oil, olive	1 tablespoon	0	120
Oil, other	1 tablespoon	0	120

RESOURCES

GRAINS AND STARCHES

	amount	grams of carbohydrate	calories
Cornstarch	1 tablespoon	7	30
Flour, all-purpose	1 tablespoon	7	28
Refried beans, traditional	1/2 cup	25	120
Holland Rusk Dry Toast	1 piece	6	30
Pepperidge Farm light bread	1 slice	9	45
Whole wheat bread	1 slice	12	70
All Bran Cereal	2 tablespoons	6	20
Oatmeal, cooked (Old Fashioned)	1 cup	27	150
Crackers, Rye Krisp	2 crackers	11	60
Harvest Bakery Multigrain Crackers	2 crackers	11	70

MISCELLANEOUS

	amount	grams of carbohydrate	calories
Beef broth, canned	1 cup	0	18
Chicken broth, canned	1 cup	1	30
Chocolate chips	1/2 cup	52	440
Chocolate syrup	2 tablespoons	24	100
Chocolate, unsweetened	1 ounce	4	95
Ice cream, chocolate	1/2 cup	19	160
Ice cream, French vanilla	1/2 cup	15	160
Brandy	1/2 cup	0	296
Sherry, dry	1 tablespoon	0	15
Wine, red	1/4 cup	0	44
Wine, white or rosé	1/2 cup	6	100
Barbeque sauce	1 tablespoon	6	25
Heinz 57 sauce	1 tablespoon	5	18
Salsa	2 tablespoons	2	10
Soy sauce	1 tablespoon	1	10
Tabasco sauce	1/4 teaspoon	0	0
Wine vinegar	1 tablespoon	1	2
Worcestershire sauce	1 teaspoon	1	5
Yellow mustard	1/2 tablespoon	0	1
Brown sugar, packed	1 tablespoon	13	51
Sugar	1 tablespoon	12	46

DAIRY PRODUCTS

	amount	grams of carbohydrate	calories
Blue cheese, crumbled	1 tablespoon	0	30
Cheddar cheese	1 ounce	0	110
Feta cheese, reduced fat, crumbled	1 tablespoon	0	15
Havarti cheese	1 ounce	0	120
Monterey Jack cheese	1 ounce	0	110
Parmesan cheese, shredded	2 tablespoons	0	55
Pepper Jack cheese	1 ounce	1	110
Swiss cheese	1 ounce	0	110
Cottage cheese, 1% fat	$1/2$ cup	5	80
Cottage cheese, 2% fat	$1/2$ cup	5	90
Cream cheese	2 tablespoons	1	100
Cream cheese, light	2 tablespoons	1	74
Cream cheese, vegetable	2 tablespoons	2	90
Cream, whipping	1 tablespoon	0	52
Milk, skim	8 ounces	12	84
Milk, 2% fat	8 ounces	12	120
Milk, whole	8 ounces	12	150
Yogurt, plain, lowfat	8 ounces	18	150

CHEESE

	grams of carbohydrate	calories
Soft Cheeses		
Brie, 1 oz.	0	95
Camembert, 1oz.	0	85
Ricotta, 1/4 cup	3	110
Cottage, 1% fat, 1/2 cup	5	80
Cream, 2 tablespoons	1	100
Semi-Soft Cheeses		
Blue, crumbled, 1 oz. (2 tablespoons)	0	60
Brick, 1 oz.	0	110
Feta, 1 oz.	0	80
Havarti, 1 oz.	0	120
Monterey Jack, 1 oz.	0	110
Mozzarella, part skim, 1 oz.	1	80
Muenster, 1 oz.	0	100
Provolone, 1 oz.	0	100
Hard Cheeses		
Cheddar, 1 oz.	0	110
Colby, 1 oz.	0	110
Edam, 1 oz.	0	90
Gouda, 1 oz.	0	110
Swiss, 1 oz.	0	110
Very Hard Cheese		
Parmesan, grated, 1 tablespoon	0	28
Parmesan, shredded, 1/4 cup	0	110
Romano, grated, 1 tablespoon	0	28
Other		
American, Pasteurized Process, 3/4 oz. slice	0	80

MY FAVORITES

	amount	grams of carbohydrate	calories

VITAMINS

Vitamin	Function	Food Sources
Vitamin A (Retinol, Beta Carotene)	• growth and repair of body tissue and immune functions • night vision * toxic in doses of 25,000 or more International Units a day)	liver, cream, butter, whole milk, egg yolk, green and yellow vegetables, yellow fruits, fortified margarine
Vitamin D (Cholecalciferol)	• calcium and phosphorus metabolism (bone & teeth formation)	fortified milk, fortified margarine, fish oils, sunlight on skin
Vitamin E (Tocopherol)	• protects cell membranes and red blood cells from oxidation • may be active in immune function	vegetable oils
Vitamin K	• formation of blood clotting agents • toxicity can be induced by water soluble analogs	cheese, egg yolk, liver, green leafy vegetables, also synthesized by intestinal bacteria
B1 (Thiamin)	• carbohydrate metabolism • appetite maintenance • nerve function • growth and muscle tone	pork, beef, liver, whole or enriched grains, legumes
B2 (Riboflavin)	• carbohydrate, fat and protein metabolism • needed for cell respiration • mucous membranes * toxic in doses above 100 milligrams a day	milk, liver, enriched cereals
Niacin	• carbohydrate, fat and protein metabolism • health of digestive system, blood circulation, nerve functioning * toxic in slow-released doses of 500 mg or more a day or immediate-release doses of 750 mg or more a day)	meat, peanuts, enriched grains
Vitamin B6 (Pyridoxine)	• carbohydrate and protein metabolism • formation of antibodies • red blood cells • nerve function	wheat, corn, meat, liver
Folate (folic acid)	• red blood cell formation • protein metabolism • cell growth and division	liver, green leafy vegetables
Vitamin C (Ascorbic Acid)	• aids wound healing, strengthens blood vessels, collagen maintenance, resistance to infection, healthy gums	citrus fruits, berries, mangos, papayas, melons, tomatoes, potatoes, green peppers and leafy green vegetables

Sources: National Academy Press, American Society for Nutritional Sciences

MINERALS

Mineral	Function	Food Sources
Calcium	• support of bones, teeth, muscle tissue • regulates heartbeat • muscle action • nerve function • blood clotting	dairy, fish (with bones), tofu, legumes, kale, broccoli, fortified foods
Chromium	• needed for glucose metabolism(energy) • increases effectiveness of insulin • muscle function	fruits, vegetables, vegetable oils, whole grains, seeds, brewer's yeast
Copper	• formation of red blood cells, pigment • needed for bone health	meat, drinking water
Iodine	• function of thyroid gland, which controls metabolism	iodized salt, bread, seafood
Iron	• formation of hemoglobin in blood and myoglobin in muscle, which supply oxygen to cells	beef, fish, poultry, shellfish, eggs, legumes, dried fruits, fortified cereals
Magnesium	• enzyme activation • nerve and muscle function • bone growth	legumes, whole grain cereals, nuts, dark green vegetables, chocolate, mineral water
Manganese	• bone growth and development • sex hormone production • cell function	non-animal sources only: fruits, vegetables, pecans, peanuts, fruit juice, oatmeal, rice
Phosphorus	• bone development • carbohydrate, fat and protein utilization	dairy, yogurt, fish, beef, poultry, eggs, legumes, grains
Potassium	• fluid balance • controls activity of heart muscle • nervous system	Fruit, vegetables, dairy, grains, legumes, beef
Selenium	• fights cell damage from oxidation	seafood, meats, grains, Brazil nuts
Sodium	• acid-base balance • fluid retention • involved in nerve impulse transmission	table salt, soy sauce, pickled foods, canned foods, many processed foods
Zinc	• taste and smell sensitivity • regulation of metabolism • aids in healing	beef, fish, poultry, grains, vegetables

Sources: National Academy Press, American Society for Nutritional Sciences

SPICY ZUCCHINI BOATS

Prep time: 20 minutes
Cook time: 12 minutes

> 4 *small zucchini*
> *Boiling, salted water*

Stuffing:
> 4 *ounces light cream cheese, softened*
> $1/2$ *cup (2 ounces) shredded pepper jack cheese*
> $1/2$ *cup shredded Parmesan cheese*
> $1/4$ *teaspoon cayenne pepper*
> 1 *teaspoon dried chives*

Preheat oven to 350 degrees. Slice zucchini in half lengthwise to make boats. Blanch zucchini in boiling, salted water, 2 minutes. Drain, then immediately immerse zucchini in an ice bath. Drain thoroughly; blot excess water with paper towels.

Using a knife or small spoon, carefully hollow out zucchini by removing some of its pulp. (Leave at least a $1/4$-inch wall.)

Combine cheeses, cayenne pepper and chives in mixing bowl. Stuff zucchini with cheese mixture. Place in lightly-greased baking dish. Bake until squash is heated through, and cheese is melted, 8 to 10 minutes.

Makes 4 (2-piece) servings.

🍎 *(per serving) Calories 210, Carbohydrates 5 gm, Protein 13 gm, Fat 16 gm, Sat Fat 7 gm, Fiber 1 gm, Cholesterol 48 mg, Sodium 476 mg*

Curves Tip: *Cover leftovers and refrigerate; reheat in microwave another day.*

(This recipe's ingredients are not included in your shopping list.)

TURKEY-LETTUCE WRAPS

Prep time: 10 minutes

8 butter lettuce leaves
$^1/_2$ cup vegetable cream cheese, softened
$^1/_2$ cucumber, peeled and diced
$^1/_4$ cup roasted and salted sunflower seeds
8 ($^1/_2$-ounce) slices deli turkey breast

Spread each lettuce leaf with 1 tablespoon cream cheese. Evenly divide cucumber and sunflower seeds between lettuce leaves and sprinkle over the cream cheese. Top each lettuce leaf with 1 slice of turkey. Press down gently and roll up.

Makes 8 wraps

● *(per wrap) Calories 80, Carbohydrates 3 gm, Protein 4 gm, Fat 6 gm, Sat Fat 3 gm, Fiber 0 gm, Cholesterol 16 mg, Sodium 179 mg*

(This recipe's ingredients are not included in your shopping list.)

ITALIAN STUFFED MUSHROOMS

Prep time: 30 minutes

$1/4$ *pound bulk Italian sausage*
$1/2$ *cup onion, minced*
  2 *cloves garlic, minced*
$1/2$ *cup zucchini, shredded*
$1/2$ *teaspoon oregano*
$1/4$ *teaspoon thyme*
  1 *teaspoon dried parsley flakes*
$1/2$ *teaspoon salt*
  3 *Rye Krisp crackers, smashed into fine crumbs (approximately $1/4$ cup)*
  2 *tablespoons shredded Parmesan cheese*
  2 *tablespoons red wine*
  2 *tablespoons water*
18 *large button mushrooms, washed*

Spray skillet with cooking spray. Brown sausage, breaking up into small crumbles as it cooks. Add onion and cook until tender. Add garlic, zucchini and spices and cook well. Turn off heat under skillet. Add crumbs, cheese, wine and water, and mix well. Remove stems from mushrooms and discard. Stuff mushroom caps with filling, piling high. Place in glass dish and cover tightly with microwave safe plastic wrap. Microwave on high power 6 to 8 minutes. Let stand 5 to 7 minutes before serving.

Makes 3 servings. (6 mushrooms each)

🍎 *(per serving) Calories 192, Carbohydrates 16 gm, Protein 9 gm, Fat 9.5 gm, Sat Fat 3 gm, Fiber 4 gm, Cholesterol 24 mg, Sodium 734 mg*

(This recipe's ingredients are not included in your shopping list.)

TUNA SALAD

Prep time: 10 minutes

1 (6-ounce) can solid white Albacore tuna (water packed)
1 green onion, minced
$^1/_2$ stalk celery, minced
1 radish, minced or shredded
$^1/_2$ teaspoon lemon juice
$^1/_2$ teaspoon lemon pepper
$^1/_2$ tablespoon yellow mustard
$1^1/_2$ tablespoons light mayonnaise

Drain tuna and break up with a fork. Add remaining ingredients and mix well.

Makes $^2/_3$ cup (1 serving)

(per serving) Calories 264, Carbohydrates 4 gm, Protein 34 gm, Fat 12.5 gm, Sat Fat 3.5 gm, Fiber 0 gm, Cholesterol 75 mg, Sodium 1309 mg

Curves Tip: Mix up enough tuna salad for the week at one time.

(This recipe's ingredients are not included in your shopping list.)

SPINACH SALAD
WITH ORANGE VINAIGRETTE

Prep time: 15 minutes

Vinaigrette:
2^1/$_2$ tablespoons orange juice
   1 tablespoon wine vinegar
1^1/$_2$ tablespoons extra-virgin or virgin olive oil
  ^{1}/$_4$ teaspoon pepper
  ^{1}/$_2$ teaspoon salt (or to taste)

Salad:
  2 cups (lightly packed) fresh spinach or baby spinach
 ^{1}/$_2$ cup sliced fresh mushrooms
 ^{1}/$_2$ cup thinly sliced red onion

For vinaigrette: Combine orange juice and vinegar in shaker.
Add oil, salt and pepper. Shake well.

For salad: Place ingredients in a serving bowl. Toss with vinaigrette to
coat vegetables.

Serve immediately.

Makes 2 servings.

🍎 *(per serving) Calories 138, Carbohydrates 11 gm, Protein 2 gm, Fat 10 gm, Sat Fat 0 gm, Fiber 2 gm, Cholesterol 0 mg, Sodium 577 mg*

(This recipe's ingredients are not included in your shopping list.)

FREE FOODS
IN THIS RECIPE:
lemon juice, lettuce,
cucumber,
red onion and garlic

*Curves dieters: 6 carbs and
348 calories per serving*

GREEK SALAD

Prep time: 20 minutes
Marinating time: at least one hour

4 ounces cooked chicken breast (no skin or breading), sliced

Dressing:
1¹/₂ tablespoons olive oil
1¹/₂ tablespoons lemon juice
1 clove garlic, mashed
¹/₂ teaspoon lemon pepper seasoning
¹/₄ teaspoon salt
¹/₄ teaspoon dried oregano
¹/₄ teaspoon dried basil

Salad:
2 cups romaine lettuce or iceberg lettuce (or mixture)
¹/₈ cucumber, sliced
¹/₂ tomato, chopped
¹/₈ cup red onion, thinly sliced
1 tablespoon sliced black olives
1 tablespoon reduced-fat feta cheese, crumbled

Whisk together dressing ingredients and pour over cooked, sliced chicken breast. Marinate in refrigerator at least one hour. Make salad and toss with chicken and dressing.

Makes 1 serving.

 (per serving) Calories 383, Carbohydrates 14 gm, Protein 29 gm, Fat 23.5 gm, Sat Fat .5 gm, Fiber 2 gm, Cholesterol 64 mg, Sodium 949 mg

(This recipe's ingredients are not included in your shopping list.)

CREAMY COLESLAW

Prep time: 10 minutes
Chilling time: 1 hour

Dressing:
  2 tablespoons heavy cream
  2 tablespoons light mayonnaise
  1 tablespoon vinegar
  $1/2$ tablespoon sugar
  $1/2$ teaspoon salt
  $1/2$ teaspoon celery seed
  $1/4$ teaspoon black pepper

  4 cups (packed) shredded cabbage (approximately 8 ounces)

  Mix dressing ingredients well. Pour over cabbage and mix. Chill until cold (at least 1 hour). The mixture will pack down to about $1^1/2$ cups.
  Makes 3 ($1/2$ cup) servings.

● (per serving) Calories 99, Carbohydrates 8 gm, Protein 0 gm, Fat 7 gm, Sat Fat 3 gm, Fiber 1 gm, Cholesterol 14 mg, Sodium 449 mg

(This recipe's ingredients are not included in your shopping list.)

FRENCH ONION SOUP

Prep time: 1 hour
Cook time: 1 hour

    4 tablespoons butter ($^1/_2$ stick)
    4 cups onions, thinly sliced (2-3 onions)
    2 cups sliced mushrooms
$1^1/_2$ tablespoons flour
    6 cups beef broth (not bouillon)
 $^1/_2$ teaspoon salt
 $^1/_2$ teaspoon pepper
 $^1/_2$ cup brandy
 $^1/_2$ teaspoon Kitchen Bouquet seasoning

On the stovetop, in a soup pot, melt the butter and add the onions, stirring constantly. Cook for 15 to 20 minutes, or until soft.

When the onions are soft, add mushrooms, cook 2 minutes and sprinkle them with flour. Stir and add 2 cups of beef broth. Continue to stir until the mixture is thickened. Add the remaining broth, and stir in salt, pepper and brandy. Bring to a boil. Cover and simmer for 45 minutes. Add the Kitchen Bouquet, and then taste for seasonings and correct if necessary.

Makes 6 ($1^1/_3$ cup) servings.

🍎 *(Per serving): Calories 199, Carbohydrates 15 gm, Protein 4 gm, Fat 8.5 gm, Sat Fat 6 gm, Fiber 3 gm, Cholesterol 21 mg, Sodium 1735 mg*

Curves Note: *Divide up into single servings and freeze until you are ready to eat.*
Curves Tip: *This soup is delicious served with 1 tablespoon shredded Parmesan cheese sprinkled on top before serving.*

(This recipe's ingredients are not included in your shopping list.)

BEEF AND VEGETABLE STEW

Prep time: 30 minutes
Cook time: 7 to 9 hours in crockpot

- 2 pounds lean beef stew meat
- 1 tablespoon olive oil
- 1 onion, sliced thinly
- 1 green pepper, julienne sliced
- 6 celery stalks, sliced
- 4 cups baby carrots
- 3 cloves garlic, minced
- 1 cup V-8 juice
- 1 teaspoon Heinz 57 steak sauce
- 1 teaspoon Worcestershire sauce
- 1/4 cup red wine
- 1/2 cup beef broth
- 1 teaspoon dried parsley flakes
- 1 tablespoon cornstarch

Brown beef in olive oil. Place meat and drippings in a large crock pot. Place vegetables on top of meat. Mix liquid ingredients and parsley and pour into crock pot. Cook on high for 7 to 9 hours. One hour before serving, mix cornstarch with 1 tablespoon water, stir until smooth. Stir into stew and mix well.

Before serving, taste and adjust seasonings, if necessary.

Makes 8 servings.

(per serving) Calories 280, Carbohydrates 13 gm, Protein 24 gm, Fat 14 gm, Sat Fat 5 gm, Fiber 3 gm, Cholesterol 60 mg, Sodium 251 mg

Curves Tip: *Freeze unused stew in single servings for later use.*

(This recipe's ingredients are not included in your shopping list.)

BEEF TENDERLOIN
WITH BLUE CHEESE

Prep and marinating time: 1 hour
Cook time: 10 to 12 minutes

    6 *(6-ounce) pieces of tenderloin, $1^1/2$ to 2 inches thick
      (2 to $2^1/2$ pounds, if buying whole tenderloin and slicing it yourself)*

Marinade:
    1 tablespoon olive oil
  $^1/4$ cup red wine
    1 clove garlic, minced
    1 tablespoon tomato paste
    1 tablespoons chopped fresh parsley
      (or 1 teaspoon dried parsley flakes)
      Salt and freshly cracked pepper to taste

$^1/2$ tablespoon blue cheese per serving

    Mix marinade ingredients in a large baking dish. Coat both sides of meat with the marinade, and let filets sit in refrigerator for 30 to 45 minutes. Grill filets over medium-high heat, or broil 6 inches from heat source, until cooked. Medium doneness is recommended (160 degrees on a meat thermometer). Top with blue cheese and cook until melted.
    Serves 6.

🍎 *(per serving) Calories 383, Carbohydrates 1 gm, Protein 38 gm, Fat 24.5 gm, Sat Fat 10 gm, Fiber 0 gm, Cholesterol 120 mg, Sodium 470 mg*

(This recipe's ingredients are not included in your shopping list.)

EASY FRITTATA

Prep time: 15 minutes

$1/2$ *pound 93% lean ground beef*
1 *tablespoon butter*
2 *cups sliced mushrooms*
$1/2$ *onion, chopped (approximately 1 cup)*
2 *teaspoons Worcestershire sauce*
1 *teaspoon dried oregano*
$1/2$ *teaspoon garlic powder*
1 *teaspoon salt*
$1/4$ *teaspoon black pepper*
1 *teaspoon dried parsley flakes*
2 *cups chopped fresh spinach*
4 *large eggs*
$1/4$ *cup skim milk*
$1/2$ *cup shredded Parmesan cheese*

Spray large skillet with nonstick cooking spray. Add ground beef, butter, mushrooms and onion; cook over medium-high heat 6 to 8 minutes or until onion is tender, breaking beef apart with spoon. Add Worcestershire sauce and seasonings. Cook until meat is no longer pink.

Stir spinach into meat mixture. Push mixture to one side of pan. Reduce heat to medium. Beat eggs with skim milk and pour into other side of pan; cook, without stirring, 1 to 2 minutes or until set on bottom. Lift eggs to allow uncooked portion to flow underneath. Repeat until softly set. Gently stir into meat mixture and heat through. Stir in cheese.

Makes 3 servings.

🍎 *(per serving) Calories 384, Carbohydrates 16 gm, Protein 33 gm, Fat 21 gm, Sat Fat 10 gm, Fiber 4 gm, Cholesterol 356 mg, Sodium 1176 mg*

(This recipe's ingredients are not included in your shopping list.)

SPICY CHILI PORK CHOPS

Prep time: 25 minutes

4 boneless pork chops (4 ounces each)

Rub:
$1/2$ *tablespoon salt*
$1/2$ *tablespoon cumin*
$1/2$ *tablespoon black pepper*
$1/2$ *tablespoon chili powder*
  1 tablespoon paprika
$1/2$ *tablespoon garlic powder*
$1/2$ *tablespoon ground ginger*

Trim fat from pork chops. Mix spices together. Rub the spice mixture into all sides of meat. Broil or grill 10 to 15 minutes on each side or until done.
Serves 4.

🍎 *(per serving) Calories 219, Carbohydrates 4 gm, Protein 19 gm, Fat 14 gm, Sat Fat 2.5 gm, Fiber 0 gm, Cholesterol 2 mg, Sodium 1652 mg*

(This recipe's ingredients are not included in your shopping list.)

FREE FOODS
IN THIS RECIPE:
**mushrooms,
green onion, garlic**

*Curves dieters: 3 carbs and
288 calories per serving*

SHERRY-MUSHROOM CHICKEN

Prep time: 45 minutes

> 3 (6 ounce) boneless, skinless chicken breasts
> 2 tablespoons olive oil
> 1^1/$_2$ cups chopped fresh mushrooms
> 2 tablespoons sliced green onion
> 1 clove garlic, minced
> 1 tablespoon cornstarch
> 1 tablespoon chopped fresh parsley or 1 teaspoon dried parsley flakes
> ^{1}/$_2$ teaspoon dried thyme
> dash black pepper
> ^{2}/$_3$ cup chicken broth
> 1 tablespoon dry sherry

In a large skillet, sauté chicken breasts in olive oil for 15 minutes or until done. When cooked, remove and keep warm in the oven while you prepare the sauce. Sauté mushrooms, green onion and garlic in skillet over medium heat until tender. Stir in cornstarch, parsley, thyme and pepper. Stir in broth and sherry. Cook and stir until sauce boils and thickens. Serve sauce over chicken.

Makes 3 servings.

🍎 *(per serving) Calories 314, Carbohydrates 8 gm, Protein 43 gm, Fat 11.5 gm, Sat Fat 1 gm, Fiber 1 gm, Cholesterol 96 gm, Sodium 113 mg*

(This recipe's ingredients are not included in your shopping list.)

JAMAICAN SEAFOOD MEDLEY

Prep time: 10 minutes
Marinating time: at least 2 hours
Cook time: 20 minutes

Marinade:
- 2 tablespoons packed brown sugar
- 1 1/2 tablespoons orange juice
- 1 1/2 tablespoons lime juice
- 2 cloves garlic, minced
- 1/2 teaspoon minced ginger
- 1 teaspoon grated orange peel
- 1 teaspoon grated lime peel
- 1 teaspoon salt
- 1/2 teaspoon black pepper
- 1/8 teaspoon ground cinnamon
- dash ground cloves
- 1/2 teaspoon Tabasco sauce

- 1/2 pound orange roughy, cut into bite-sized pieces
- 1/2 pound sea scallops, cut in half (or quarters, if very large)
- 1/2 pound shrimp, shelled and deveined
- 1 tablespoon olive oil
- 3/4 cup baby corn, snapped in fourths
- 1 tablespoon green onions, sliced
- 1/2 green pepper, julienne sliced

Combine sugar, juices and seasonings. Pour over seafood; mix well.
Cover and refrigerate at least 2 hours. Drain seafood and discard
marinade. Saute seafood and vegetables in olive oil over medium heat
for 15 minutes or until done. Serves 3.

🍎 *(per serving) Calories 287, Carbohydrates 7 gm, Protein 41 gm, Fat 10.5 gm, Sat Fat 0.5 gm,
Fiber 2 gm, Cholesterol 156 mg, Sodium 433 mg*

(This recipe's ingredients are not included in your shopping list.)

TOFU STIR-FRY

Prep time: 15 minutes

3 ounces firm tofu ($^1/_5$ block)
2 tablespoons olive oil
$^1/_2$ onion, thinly sliced
1 clove garlic, chopped
$^1/_2$ cup mushrooms, sliced
$^1/_2$ cup zucchini, sliced
$^1/_2$ cup fresh spinach, packed
1 tablespoon soy sauce
1 tablespoon water

Press water from tofu by putting between several layers of paper towels and placing a dinner plate on top. Let sit 20 to 30 minutes. Divide block into 5 portions. (*The 4 unused portions of tofu may be frozen in individual bags for later use.*)

Cube tofu and stir fry in olive oil. Add onion and garlic and cook 3 to 4 minutes. Add mushrooms and cook until done. Add zucchini and cook a few minutes. Add spinach, soy sauce and water. Stir well and cook 1 to 2 minutes.

Serves 1.

● *(Per serving): Calories 440, Carbohydrates 25 gm, Protein 12 gm, Fat 31.5 gm, Sat Fat 1 gm, Fiber 4 gm, Cholesterol 0 mg, Sodium 987 mg*

Curves Tip: *3 ounces of chicken can be substituted for tofu. (Nutritional information remains approximately the same.)*

(This recipe's ingredients are not included in your shopping list.)

PARMESAN VEGETABLE STIR-FRY

Prep time: 15 minutes

1 tablespoon olive oil
$^1/_2$ onion, thinly sliced
1 clove garlic, chopped
$^1/_2$ cup mushrooms, sliced
1 cup fresh spinach
1 tablespoon lemon juice
$^1/_2$ ounce (2 tablespoons) Parmesan cheese, shredded

Sauté onion and garlic in olive oil until soft. Add mushrooms and cook until done. Add spinach, toss well and sauté very briefly. Sprinkle on lemon juice and Parmesan cheese. Serve hot.

Makes 1 serving.

● *(per serving) Calories 275, Carbohydrates 22 gm, Protein 8 gm, Fat 17 gm, Sat Fat 0 gm, Fiber 6 gm, Cholesterol 10 mg, Sodium 1189 mg*

(This recipe's ingredients are not included in your shopping list.)

FROZEN CHOCOLATE MOUSSE

Prep time: 30 minutes
Freezing time: at least 1 hour

12 ounces silken (soft) tofu
$^1/_2$ cup semisweet chocolate chips
$1^1/_2$ ounces unsweetened chocolate
$^1/_2$ cup Splenda (granular)
$^1/_4$ cup water
3 egg whites
$^1/_4$ teaspoon salt
2 tablespoons heavy cream
1 teaspoon vanilla extract

Remove tofu from water in package and place between several layers of paper towels. Weight with a plate for at least 15 minutes to press excess water out of tofu.

Place chocolate chips and unsweetened chocolate in a microwave-proof bowl. Cover and microwave 1 minute, or until melted. Stir well and set aside. Combine Splenda and water in a small saucepan and bring to a boil. Turn off heat under saucepan. In a medium bowl, beat egg whites and salt on high speed until stiff peaks form. Continue beating on high and pour hot syrup very slowly into beaten egg whites. Set meringue aside.

Beat tofu, melted chocolate, heavy cream, and vanilla until very smooth. Beat in half of meringue. Fold in remaining meringue. Line 8 cupcake pan wells with paper cupcake liners. Spoon approximately $^1/_4$ cup of mousse into each and pack down well. Cover with plastic wrap and freeze about 1 hour. Remove from cupcake pan (you may need to rub the bottom of the pan with a hot, wet washcloth to free the liner) and put into a freezer bag. Store in freezer until ready to serve.

Before serving, let frozen mousse sit at room temperature for 5 minutes before peeling off paper liner.

Makes 8 ($^1/_4$ cup) servings.

🍎 (per serving) Calories 127, Carbohydrates 9 gm, Protein 7 gm, Fat 7 gm, Sat Fat 1 gm, Fiber 1 gm, Cholesterol 5 mg, Sodium 161

Curves Note: For a more traditional mousse, this recipe may be chilled in the refrigerator for at least 2 hours instead of freezing in a cupcake pan.

Curves Tip: To vary the taste of this dessert, use other flavorings instead of vanilla extract, such as 1 teaspoon orange extract or 1 tablespoon creme de menthe liqueur.

(This recipe's ingredients are not included in your shopping list.)

I'M READY FOR THE CURVES DIET
CHECKLIST

_____I have taken the tests on pages 28 and 29 to determine which diet plan I should follow

_____I have tried the Curves shake and I know I can drink it every day

_____I have a blender or shaker to make the Curves shake

_____I have bought the Curves shake

_____I can drink 8 (8-ounce) glasses of water per day

_____I know how to weigh and measure foods

_____I have access to *The Complete Book of Food Counts* book by Corinne T. Netzer or something like it

_____I know how to look up the calorie and carbohydrate counts of food

_____I have made sure I have all the foods on the shopping list on page 76, the foods on the Free Foods List (page 31), and the pantry essentials on page 34

_____I have met with my Curves instructor to discuss my diet plan

_____I have gone to Curves to have my beginning weight, body fat and measurements taken and I have recorded them in the charts on pages 25 and 26.

Vegetables
____ 1/2 cup asparagus
____ 1 cup broccoli florets
____ 1 cup brussels sprouts
____ 1/2 cup carrots, baby
____ 1 1/2 cup cauliflower florets
____ 1 stalk celery
____ 1/2 cup green beans
____ 2 green onions
____ 1/2 cup mushrooms, sliced
____ 1/2 cup onion
____ *2 tomatoes, small
____ 1/2 cup zucchini, sliced

_____
_____
_____

Free Foods
____ enough for 7 salads

Dairy
____ 4 tablespoons butter
____ 2 ounces Cheddar cheese
____ 2 1/2 cups cottage cheese, lowfat (1%), small curd
____ 4 eggs
____ 4 ounces Havarti cheese
____ 1/2 gallon milk, skim
____ 1/2 ounce Parmesan cheese, shredded (2 tablespoons)
____ 8 ounces yogurt, plain, lowfat

_____
_____

Fruit
____ *1 small apple
____ *2 tablespoons blueberries
____ 1 1/2 cup cantaloupe, cubed
____ *1 grapefruit
____ *1 medium orange
____ *1 peach
____ 1 cup strawberries

_____

Meat and Seafood
____ 24 ounces chicken breast (divided)
____ 6-ounce pork chop, lean
____ 10 ounces ground beef, 93% lean (divided)
____ 4-ounce sirloin steak, well trimmed
____ 4 ounces roast beef, deli
____ 2 ounces turkey breast, deli
____ 8 ounces ham, lean (divided)
____ 4 slices bacon
____ 6 breakfast sausage links
____ 8 ounces orange roughy
____ 8 ounces salmon
____ 8 ounces shrimp, peeled
____ 1 (3-ounce) can solid white albacore tuna, packed in water

_____

Starches
____ *4 Keebler Harvest Bakery Multigrain Crackers
____ *2 Rye Krisp Crackers
____ 2 slices whole wheat bread

_____

Other
____ 2 tablespoons mayonnaise
____ 1 tablespoon peanut butter
____ *1 ounce dry roasted peanuts
____ *8 ounces V-8 juice

Recipes this week
____ Easy Frittata, page 68
____ French Onion Soup, page 65
____ Parmesan Vegetable Stir-Fry, page 73
____ Tuna Salad, page 61

*If you are following the carbohydrate-restricted version, you will not be eating the foods marked with an asterisk, so don't buy them.

PHASE I

Take the tests on pages 28 & 29 to determine whether you are a candidate for the higher protein dieting advantage or whether you should follow the calorie-restricted method.

~

HIGHER PROTEIN/LOW CARBOHYDRATE

For the higher protein/low carbohydrate version, you should:

Enjoy unlimited amounts of lean meats, cheeses, eggs, seafood and poultry
(baked, broiled, or boiled—never fried).

Eat moderate to lower amounts of fat.

Limit your carbohydrate intake to 20 grams per day
(not counting free foods).

Eat, but don't cheat!

If you do not feel that you have adequate energy with this version or if you
have not lost weight after a few days, switch to the calorie-restricted method.

CALORIE-RESTRICTED

For the calorie-restricted version, you should:

Eat no more than 1200 calories per day (not counting free foods).

Consume 40% of those calories in the form of protein foods.

Consume no more than 60 grams of carbohydrates per day (not counting free foods).

~

With either plan you may enjoy one Curves shake per day
and unlimited amounts of free foods.

Be sure to drink 8 glasses of water daily and take a good multi-vitamin & mineral supplement.

*You will follow Phase I for 1 or 2 weeks. If you have less than 20 pounds to lose you may
move to Phase II after 1 week. If you have 20 or more pounds to lose, you will follow Phase I for 2 weeks.*

> **HINT:** You are not required to eat the meals in the order they are listed.
> Feel free to adjust them to your lifestyle and schedule.

EMBRACING CHANGE

Change is difficult, even change that will have a positive impact on our lives. For any change of habits to have a chance to take root, we must have a plan of action. Jumping into change for emotional reasons is not likely to produce a lasting effect.

In order to get through the pain of dealing with change, you must become comfortable with being uncomfortable. You must believe that the change is for the better, and that it will not always involve the difficulty that it now does. You must be willing to look for bright spots in the midst of what seems like misery.

You can succeed. You have done more difficult things than this, and you have what it takes to follow this plan for six weeks.

List 5 reasons to lose weight:
1. _____
2. _____
3. _____
4. _____
5. _____

List 2 things that will be great about doing this 6-week challenge:
1. _____
   _____
2. _____
   _____

List 4 fears you have about undertaking this challenge :
1. . _____
2. _____
3. _____
4. _____

GOALS

Setting realistic and measurable goals is one way of keeping your motivation high through this 6-week challenge. Here is an example of a goal that is not helpful:

a 60 year old woman who is 5 feet tall and weighs 175 pounds wants to look like a super model

This goal is unrealistic because many super models are only seventeen years old and nearly six feet tall. In addition, this goal is not measurable. A much more helpful set of goals for that fictional woman might be to lose 10-15 pounds of body fat, to work out three times a week, to drink 64 oz. of water every day, and to take a multi-vitamin every day.

Even a seemingly-reasonable goal such as "I want to feel better" is not measurable, and is therefore not a helpful goal. Try to name specific ways you want to feel better (fewer headaches, fewer backaches, fewer upset stomachs, etc.) and attempt to quantify them.

List 8 of your goals:
1. _____
2. _____
3. _____
4. _____
5. _____
6. _____
7. _____
8. _____

Which 2 of your goals are not realistic?
1. _____
2. _____

Which 2 of your goals are not measurable?
1. _____
2. _____

Do you want to set some new goals for yourself? _____
_____
_____
_____

"Do you not know that your body is a temple
of the Holy Spirit, who is in you,
whom you have received from God?

1 Corinthians 6:19

Goals for Monday:

Physical: _____
_____
_____

Mental: _____
_____
_____

Spiritual: _____
_____
_____

What do I hope to change by being on this diet? What are my goals for this diet? _____
_____
_____
_____
_____

What am I thankful for today? _____
_____
_____

One nice thing I've done for myself today... _____
_____
_____
_____
_____
_____
_____

Day: Monday

		Carbs	Calories
Meal 1	¹/₂ cup 1% fat cottage cheese	5	80
	¹/₂ cup strawberries	6	23
Meal 2	Curves shake with 8 oz. skim milk	FREE	FREE
Meal 3	4 ounces 93% lean ground beef, broiled	0	160
	Free Foods Salad		
	Salad Dressing (your choice)		
Meal 4	²/₃ cup tuna salad (recipe page 61)	3	258
	*2 Rye Krisp crackers	11	60
Meal 5	6 ounces chicken breast, broiled	0	186
	Parmesan Vegetable Stir Fry (recipe page 73)	0	175
Meal 6	3 ounces lean ham	0	100
	*1 small apple	20	80

Water: ▯ ▯ ▯ ▯ ▯ ▯ ▯ ▯

Vitamins: ▭ ▭ ▭

Totals for Day	1122

Today's Exercise:

Curves Workout ♡

or

Aerobic ♡

_____

_____

Strength Training ♡

_____

_____

Stretching ♡

_____

_____

Go to Curves today to be weighed, measured and have your body fat tested. Record your beginning weight, body fat, and measurements on the charts on pages 25 and 26.

If you are following the carbohydrate-restricted version, don't eat the foods that are marked with an asterisk (*). You should eat larger quantities of no-carb foods than this food diary specifies in order to get enough calories.

PHASE I

"I'm just a person trapped inside a woman's body."

—Elayne Boosler

Goals for Tuesday:

Physical: _____

_____

_____

Mental: _____

_____

Spiritual: _____

_____

_____

Do I have certain genetic traits that cannot be changed by improving my eating or exercise habits? (i.e. height, bust size, bone size, shoe size, etc.) _____

_____

_____

_____

_____

_____

_____

_____

_____

What am I thankful for today? _____

_____

_____

One nice thing I've done for myself today... _____

_____

_____

Day: Tuesday

		Carbs	Calories
Meal 1	2 ounces Deli turkey breast	2	60
	*1 sliced tomato	6	30
	1/2 slice whole wheat bread	6	35
	1 tablespoon mayonnaise	0	100
Meal 2	1/2 cup cubed cantaloupe	6	25
	1/2 cup 1% fat cottage cheese	5	80
Meal 3	6 ounces chicken breast, broiled	0	186
	Free Foods Salad		
	Salad Dressing (your choice)		
Meal 4	Curves shake with 8 oz. skim milk	FREE	FREE
Meal 5	4 ounces sirloin steak, broiled	0	215
	1/2 cup steamed broccoli	FREE	FREE
	1/2 cup steamed cauliflower	FREE	FREE
	1 tablespoon butter	0	102
Meal 6	1 ounce Havarti cheese	0	120
	*1 ounce dry roasted peanuts	5	160

Water: ⬜ ⬜ ⬜ ⬜ ⬜ ⬜ ⬜
Vitamins: ⬭ ⬭ ⬭

Totals for Day

Today's Exercise:

Curves Workout ♡

or

Aerobic ♡

_____
_____

Strength Training ♡

_____
_____

Stretching ♡

_____
_____

If you are following the carbohydrate-restricted version, don't eat the foods that are marked with an asterisk (*). You should eat larger quantities of no-carb foods than this food diary specifies in order to get enough calories.

PHASE I

"He loves each one of us
as if there were only one of us"
—*Augustine*

Goals for Wednesday:

Physical: _____
_____
_____

Mental: _____
_____
_____

Spiritual: _____
_____
_____

Do I believe my body is good and worthy of being treated as
a creation of God? _____
_____
_____
_____
_____
_____
_____
_____

What am I thankful for today? _____
_____
_____

One nice thing I've done for myself today... _____
_____
_____

Day: Wednesday

			Carbs	Calories
Meal 1		1 serving Easy Frittata (recipe page 68)	4	325
		*1 peach	9	37
Meal 2		Curves shake with 8 oz. skim milk	FREE	FREE
Meal 3		4 ounces Deli roast beef	4	120
		Free Foods Salad		
		Salad Dressing (your choice)		
Meal 4		4 ounces plain yogurt	9	75
		*2 tablespoons blueberries	4	14
Meal 5		6 ounces broiled pork chop	0	225
		1/2 cup zucchini sautéed in:	FREE	FREE
		1/2 tablespoon olive oil	0	60
Meal 6		2 ounces lean ham	0	67
		2 ounces Cheddar cheese	0	220

Water: ⊓ ⊓ ⊓ ⊓ ⊓ ⊓ ⊓ ⊓

Vitamins: ⊖ ⊖ ⊖

Totals for Day

Today's Exercise:

Curves Workout ♡

or

Aerobic ♡

_____

_____

Strength Training ♡

_____

_____

Stretching ♡

_____

_____

If you are following the carbohydrate-restricted version, don't eat the foods that are marked with an asterisk (*). You should eat larger quantities of no-carb foods than this food diary specifies in order to get enough calories.

"Life itself is the proper binge."

—*Julia Child*

Goals for Thursday:

Physical: _____
_____
_____

Mental: _____
_____
_____

Spiritual: _____
_____
_____

Can I name any eating habits that undermine my ability to eat moderately and healthy? (i.e. binge eating, eating in secret, skipping meals, excessive sugar, salt or fatty-food cravings, etc.) _____
_____
_____
_____
_____
_____
_____
_____

What am I thankful for today? _____
_____
_____

One nice thing I've done for myself today... _____
_____
_____

Day: Thursday

		Carbs	Calories
Meal 1	4 slices bacon	0	120
	$^{1}/_{2}$ slice whole wheat bread	6	35
	1 tablespoon mayonnaise	0	100
	*1 tomato, sliced	6	30
Meal 2	$^{1}/_{2}$ cup 1% fat cottage cheese	5	80
	$^{1}/_{2}$ cup baby carrots	5	24
Meal 3	3 ounces water-packed tuna	0	90
	Free Foods Salad		
	Salad Dressing (your choice)		
Meal 4	Curves shake with 8 oz. skim milk	FREE	FREE
Meal 5	Stir Fry of:		
	1 tablespoon olive oil	0	120
	8 ounces chicken breast	0	248
	$^{1}/_{2}$ cup onion	FREE	FREE
	$^{1}/_{2}$ cup mushrooms	FREE	FREE
	$^{1}/_{2}$ cup asparagus	FREE	FREE
Meal 6	2 ounces Havarti cheese	0	240
	*1 medium orange	16	65

Water: ⊔ ⊔ ⊔ ⊔ ⊔ ⊔ ⊔ ⊔

Vitamins: ⊐ ⊐ ⊐

Totals for Day

Today's Exercise:

Curves Workout ♡

or

Aerobic ♡

_____

_____

Strength Training ♡

_____

_____

Stretching ♡

_____

_____

PHASE I

If you are following the carbohydrate-restricted version, don't eat the foods that are marked with an asterisk (*). You should eat larger quantities of no-carb foods than this food diary specifies in order to get enough calories.

Live in harmony with one another.

Romans 12:16

PHASE I

Goals for Friday:

Physical: _____

_____

_____

Mental: _____

_____

_____

Spiritual: _____

_____

_____

What areas of my life are out of balance? _____

_____

_____

_____

_____

_____

_____

_____

_____

_____

What am I thankful for today? _____

_____

_____

One nice thing I've done for myself today... _____

_____

_____

_____

_____

Day: Friday

		Carbs	Calories
Meal 1	3 ounces lean ham	0	100
	2 eggs	0	150
	*1/2 grapefruit	12	46
Meal 2	1/2 cup 1% fat cottage cheese	5	80
	1/2 cup cubed cantaloupe	6	25
Meal 3	8 ounces broiled salmon	0	414
	1 cup brussels sprouts	FREE	FREE
	1 tablespoon butter	0	102
Meal 4	Curves shake with 8 oz. skim milk	FREE	FREE
Meal 5	Free Foods Salad		
	2 tablespoons shredded Parmesan cheese	0	55
	Salad Dressing (your choice)		
Meal 6	1 stalk celery	FREE	FREE
	1 tablespoon peanut butter	4	95
	*2 Keebler Harvest Bakery Multigrain Crackers	11	70

Water: 🥛🥛🥛🥛🥛🥛🥛

Vitamins: ⬭ ⬭ ⬭

Totals for Day		

Today's Exercise:

Curves Workout ♡

or

Aerobic ♡

_____

_____

Strength Training ♡

_____

_____

Stretching ♡

_____

_____

If you are following the carbohydrate-restricted version, don't eat the foods that are marked with an asterisk (*). You should eat larger quantities of no-carb foods than this food diary specifies in order to get enough calories.

*Why are you downcast, O my soul? Why so
disturbed within me? Put your hope in God,
for I will yet praise him, my Savior and my God.*

Psalm 42:5

PHASE I

Goals for Saturday:

Physical: _____
_____
_____

Mental: _____
_____
_____

Spiritual: _____
_____
_____

Do I eat when I'm bored, tired, sad, mad or stressed? _____
_____
_____
_____
_____
_____
_____

What am I thankful for today? _____
_____
_____

One nice thing I've done for myself today... _____
_____
_____
_____

Day: Saturday

		Carbs	Calories
Meal 1	¹/₂ slice whole wheat bread	6	35
	1 ounce Havarti cheese	0	120
	3 sausage links	0	200
Meal 2	Curves shake with 8 oz. skim milk	FREE	FREE
Meal 3	Free Foods Salad		
	Salad Dressing (your choice)		
Meal 4	6 ounces 93% hamburger, broiled	0	240
	*8 ounces V-8 juice	10	46
Meal 5	8 ounces shrimp, broiled	0	240
	1 serving French Onion Soup (recipe page 65)	3	145
	¹/₂ cup broccoli, steamed	FREE	FREE
	1 teaspoon butter	0	34
Meal 6	4 ounces plain yogurt	9	75
	*¹/₂ cup strawberries	6	23

Water: 🥛🥛🥛🥛🥛🥛🥛

Vitamins: 💊 💊 💊

Totals for Day

Today's Exercise:

Curves Workout ♡

or

Aerobic ♡

_____

_____

Strength Training ♡

_____

_____

Stretching ♡

_____

_____

PHASE I

If you are following the carbohydrate-restricted version, don't eat the foods that are marked with an asterisk (*). You should eat larger quantities of no-carb foods than this food diary specifies in order to get enough calories.

"Nothing in life is to be feared,
it is only to be understood."

—*Marie Curie*

Goals for Sunday:

Physical: _____

_____

_____

Mental: _____

_____

_____

Spiritual: _____

_____

_____

What do I fear most about being fat? _____

_____

_____

What do I fear most about being thin? _____

_____

_____

What am I thankful for today? _____

_____

_____

One nice thing I've done for myself today... _____

_____

_____

_____

Day: Sunday

		Carbs	Calories
Meal 1	2 eggs	0	150
	3 sausage links	0	200
	*1/2 grapefruit	12	46
Meal 2	4 ounces chicken breast, broiled	0	124
	1/2 cup green beans	4	20
	1 teaspoon butter	0	34
Meal 3	Free Foods Salad		
	Salad Dressing (your choice)		
Meal 4	1/2 cup 1% fat cottage cheese	5	80
	1/2 cup cubed cantaloupe	6	25
	*2 Keebler Harvest Bakery Multigrain Crackers	11	70
Meal 5	8 ounces orange roughy sautéed in:	0	216
	1 tablespoon olive oil	0	120
	1 cup steamed cauliflower	FREE	FREE
	1/2 tablespoon butter	0	51
Meal 6	Curves shake with 8 oz. skim milk	FREE	FREE

Water: 🥛🥛🥛🥛🥛🥛🥛🥛

Vitamins: ⬭ ⬭ ⬭

Totals for Day

PHASE I

93

SHOPPING LIST–PHASE II, WEEK 1

(If you have another week on Phase I,
use the shopping list on page 76)

Vegetables
____1 cup asparagus
____1 cup broccoli florets
____1 cup green beans
____1 cup mushrooms, sliced
____1/2 cup onion
____2 cups spinach, fresh
____1 tomato, small
____2 cups zucchini, sliced

_____

Free Foods
____enough for 5 salads

Dairy
____2 tablespoons butter
____5 ounces Cheddar cheese
____1 1/2 cups cottage cheese,
     lowfat (1%), small curd
____5 eggs
____5 ounces Havarti cheese
____1/2 gallon milk, skim
____2 tablespoons vegetable
     cream cheese
____12 ounces yogurt, plain,
     lowfat

_____

Fruit
____1 small apple
____1 banana
____1/4 cup blueberries
____1 cup cantaloupe, cubed
____1 cup seedless grapes
____1 medium orange
____1 peach
____1 cup strawberries

_____

Meat
____36 ounces chicken breast
     (divided)
____8-ounce pork chop, lean
____6-ounce sirloin steak, well
     trimmed

____12 ounces ground beef,
     93% lean (divided)
____7 ounces ham, lean (divided)
____6 breakfast sausage links
____4 slices bacon
____8 ounces shrimp
____8 ounces salmon

_____

Starches
____4 Keebler Harvest Bakery
     Multigrain crackers
____6 Rye Krisp Crackers
____2 slices whole wheat bread

_____

Other
____2 ounces roasted and salted
     almonds
____1 ounce roasted and salted
     cashews
____2 ounces pistachio nuts,
     in shells
____2 tablespoons peanut butter
____1/2 cup refried beans
____2 tablespoons salsa
____16 ounces V-8 juice

_____

Recipes this week
____Beef and Vegetable Stew,
     page 66
____Beef Tenderloin with Blue
     Cheese, page 67
____French Onion Soup, page 65
____Parmesan Vegetable Stir-Fry,
     page 73
____Spicy Zucchini Boats,
     page 58
____Spinach Salad, page 62
____Tofu Stir-Fry, page 72
____Tuna Salad, page 61
____Turkey-Lettuce Wraps,
     page 59

PHASE I
~ WEEK 2 ~

If you are beginning your second week of Phase I, use the shopping list on page 76. Your food plan is in bold in the following food diaries. You should expect to lose about 2-3 pounds during the second week of Phase I.

~

PHASE II
~ WEEK 1 ~

If you began with less than 20 pounds to lose, you have completed Phase I. You may now move to Phase II, which has a larger amount and variety of food. Use the shopping list on page 94. You should expect to lose 1-2 pounds per week during Phase II. If you are following the higher protein/low carbohydrate method be prepared to switch to the calorie version if:
- *During Phase I, week 1, you lost less than 3 pounds*
- *During Phase I, week 2, you lose less than 2 pounds*
- *During Phase II, any week, you lose less than 1 pound*

~

HIGHER PROTEIN/LOW CARBOHYDRATE

For the higher protein/low carbohydrate version, you should:

Enjoy unlimited amounts of lean meats, cheeses, eggs, seafood and poultry (baked, broiled, or boiled—never fried).

Eat moderate to lower amounts of fat.

Limit your carbohydrate intake to 40-60 grams per day (not counting free foods).

Eat, but don't cheat!

CALORIE-RESTRICTED

For the calorie-restricted version, you should:

Eat no more than 1600 calories per day (not counting free foods).

Consume 40% of those calories in the form of protein foods.

Consume no more than 60 grams of carbohydrates per day (not counting free foods).

~

HINT: You are not required to eat the meals in the order they are listed. Feel free to adjust them to your lifestyle and schedule.

DIETS DON'T WORK

PHASE II - 1

List 3 dieting methods you have tried:

1. _____

2. _____

3. _____

List 2 dieting methods that have worked for you on a short-term basis:

1. _____

   _____

2. _____

   _____

Name a dieting method that has worked for you and helped you maintain your results for at least 2 years:

_____

_____

_____

_____

Restricting calories causes a decrease in metabolic rate. So why do other diets require us to continue to limit caloric intake?

Don't they know that hormones are produced in response to dieting which allow the body to operate more efficiently? The body is trying to protect us from losing fat, because it doesn't know the difference between intentional dieting and starvation due to famine or disaster. And so, weight loss slows and a plateau is reached on any diet.

When this happens, other diets require us to limit our calories even further. We cannot get ahead of this vicious cycle. Furthermore, so-called maintenance programs are really perpetual diets. Since we now know that perpetual dieting perpetuates a low metabolism, we don't need to feel badly about past failed diets. The problem was not our lack of willpower, the problem was a decreased metabolic rate.

THE CHALLENGE

This 6 week challenge will give you the opportunity to try foods you may have avoided in the past. You may even learn to like some new foods. It will also give you the opportunity to break your addiction to carbohydrates. You should expect to feel remarkably better within the first two weeks. However, you may experience headaches, nausea, and fatigue as your body adjusts to this new way of eating. Don't worry—these symptoms should go away. Drink plenty of water, continue exercising, take your vitamins, and get enough sleep to help yourself through the adjustment period. If you do not feel well on the higher protein/low carbohydrate version, switch to the calorie method.

Some women complain that the daily menu plans contain too much food. Be realistic—you obviously have been eating a lot more food than this on a regular basis, or you wouldn't have a weight problem. Perhaps you are put off by eating more protein. Keep trying and remember that it took time for your body to grow accustomed to the way you used to eat.

Give yourself time to adjust.

Make a list of the 5 hardest things about this 6 week challenge.
1._____
2._____
3._____
4._____
5._____

Make a list of 5 foods you must give up during this 6 week challenge.
1._____
2._____
3._____
4._____
5._____

Make a list of 5 foods you will enjoy eating during this 6 week challenge.
1._____
2._____
3._____
4._____
5._____

He will yet fill your mouth with laughter
and your lips with shouts of joy.

Job 8:21

Goals for Monday:

Physical: _____

_____

_____

Mental: _____

_____

_____

Spiritual: _____

_____

_____

When was the last time I laughed really hard? _____

_____

_____

_____

_____

_____

_____

What am I thankful for today? _____

_____

_____

One nice thing I've done for myself today... _____

_____

_____

_____

_____

Day: Monday

		Carbs	Calories
Meal 1	1/2 cup 1% fat cottage cheese	5	80
	1 cup seedless grapes	28	114
	1/2 cup 1% fat cottage cheese	**5**	**80**
	1/2 cup strawberries	**6**	**23**
Meal 2	Curves shake with 8 oz. skim milk	FREE	FREE
	Curves shake with 8 oz. skim milk	**FREE**	**FREE**
Meal 3	6 ounces 93% lean ground beef, broiled	0	240
	1 serving French Onion Soup (recipe page 65)	3	145
	Free Foods Salad		
	Salad Dressing (your choice)		
	4 ounces 93% lean ground beef, broiled	**0**	**160**
	Free Foods Salad		
	Salad Dressing (your choice)		
Meal 4	2/3 cup tuna salad (recipe page 61)	3	258
	2 Rye Krisp crackers	11	60
	2/3 cup tuna salad (recipe page 61)	**3**	**258**
	***2 Rye Krisp crackers**	**11**	**60**
Meal 5	8 ounces chicken breast, broiled	0	248
	Parmesan Vegetable Stir Fry (recipe page 73)	0	175
	4 ounces V-8 juice	5	23
	6 ounces chicken breast, broiled	**0**	**186**
	Parmesan Vegetable Stir Fry		
	(recipe page 73)	**0**	**175**
Meal 6	2 ounces lean ham	0	67
	1 ounce Havarti cheese	0	120
	3 ounces lean ham	**0**	**100**
	***1 small apple**	**20**	**80**

Water: ⛢⛢⛢⛢⛢⛢⛢⛢

Vitamins: ⬭⬭⬭

Totals for Day

Today's Exercise:

Curves Workout ♡

or

Aerobic ♡

_____

_____

Strength Training ♡

_____

_____

Stretching ♡

_____

_____

Today you need to go to Curves to be weighed and have your body fat tested. Record your results here:

Weight_____
% Body Fat _____
Pounds of
Body Fat _____

Also record your results on the chart on page 26.

If you are doing the 2nd week of Phase I, you need to eat the foods in bold print.

If you are following the carbohydrate-restricted version, don't eat the foods that are marked with an asterisk (*). You should eat larger quantities of no-carb foods than this food diary specifies.

*"If you follow your bliss...the life that you ought
to be living is the one you are living."*

—Joseph Campbell

Goals for Tuesday:

Physical: _____
_____

Mental: _____
_____

Spiritual: _____
_____
_____

Do I live in the moment or am I constantly worried about the
past or future? _____
_____
_____
_____
_____
_____
_____

What am I thankful for today? _____
_____
_____

One nice thing I've done for myself today... _____
_____
_____
_____

Day: Tuesday

		Carbs	Calories
Meal 1	2 eggs	0	150
	1 sliced tomato	6	30
	2 ounces Deli turkey breast	**2**	**60**
	***1 sliced tomato**	**6**	**30**
	1/2 slice whole wheat bread	**6**	**35**
	1 tablespoon mayonnaise	**0**	**100**
Meal 2	1/2 cup cubed cantaloupe	6	25
	1/2 cup 1% fat cottage cheese	5	80
	1 ounce roasted and salted almonds	4	180
	1/2 cup cubed cantaloupe	**6**	**25**
	1/2 cup 1% fat cottage cheese	**5**	**80**
Meal 3	6 ounces chicken breast, broiled	0	186
	Free Foods Salad		
	Salad Dressing (your choice)		
	6 ounces chicken breast, broiled	**0**	**186**
	Free Foods Salad		
	Salad Dressing (your choice)		
Meal 4	Curves shake with 8 oz. skim milk	FREE	FREE
	Curves shake with 8 oz. skim milk	**FREE**	**FREE**
Meal 5	8 ounces broiled salmon	0	414
	1 cup steamed broccoli	FREE	FREE
	1/2 tablespoon butter	0	51
	4 ounces sirloin steak, broiled	**0**	**215**
	1/2 cup steamed broccoli	**FREE**	**FREE**
	1/2 cup steamed cauliflower	**FREE**	**FREE**
	1 tablespoon butter	**0**	**102**
Meal 6	2 ounces Havarti cheese	0	240
	2 Rye Krisp crackers	11	60
	1 small apple	20	80
	1 ounce Havarti cheese	**0**	**120**
	***1 ounce dry roasted peanuts**	**5**	**160**

Water: 🥛🥛🥛🥛🥛🥛🥛

Vitamins: ⬭ ⬭ ⬭

Totals for Day

Today's Exercise:

Curves Workout ♡

or

Aerobic ♡

_____

Strength Training ♡

_____

_____

Stretching ♡

_____

_____

If you are doing the 2nd week of Phase I, you need to eat the foods in bold print.

If you are following the carbohydrate-restricted version, don't eat the foods that are marked with an asterisk (*). You should eat larger quantities of no-carb foods than this food diary specifies.

For I am the Lord, your God,
who takes hold of your right hand and says to you:
Do not fear; I will help you.

Isaiah 41:13

Goals for Wednesday:

Physical: _____

_____

_____

Mental: _____

_____

_____

Spiritual: _____

_____

_____

Is there any significant person in my life who does not
support my efforts to change? _____

_____

_____

_____

_____

_____

What am I thankful for today? _____

_____

_____

One nice thing I've done for myself today... _____

_____

_____

_____

Day: <u>Wednesday</u>

		Carbs	Calories
Meal 1	8 ounces plain yogurt	18	150
	1/4 cup blueberries	7	27
	1 serving Easy Frittata (recipe page 68)	**4**	**325**
	***1 peach**	**9**	**37**
Meal 2	Curves shake with 8 oz. skim milk	FREE	FREE
	Curves shake with 8 oz. skim milk	**FREE**	**FREE**
Meal 3	1 serving Spinach Salad (page 62)		
	with 2 tablespoons Orange Vinaigrette	3	101
	8 ounces chicken breast, broiled	0	248
	4 ounces Deli roast beef	**4**	**120**
	Free Foods Salad		
	Salad Dressing (your choice)		
Meal 4	2/3 cup tuna salad (recipe page 61)	3	258
	2 Rye Krisp Crackers	11	60
	8 ounces V-8 juice	10	46
	4 ounces plain yogurt	**9**	**75**
	***2 tablespoons blueberries**	**4**	**14**
Meal 5	6 ounces broiled sirloin steak	0	323
	1 cup zucchini sautéed in:	FREE	FREE
	1 tablespoon olive oil	0	120
	6 ounces broiled pork chop	**0**	**225**
	1/2 cup zucchini sautéed in:	**FREE**	**FREE**
	1/2 tablespoon olive oil	**0**	**60**
Meal 6	3 ounces lean ham	0	100
	1 ounce Havarti cheese	0	120
	2 ounces lean ham	**0**	**67**
	2 ounces Cheddar cheese	**0**	**220**

Water: 🥛🥛🥛🥛🥛🥛🥛 Totals for Day

Vitamins: ⬭ ⬭ ⬭

Today's Exercise:

Curves Workout ♡

or

Aerobic ♡

_____

_____

Strength Training ♡

_____

_____

Stretching ♡

_____

_____

If you are doing the 2nd week of Phase I, you need to eat the foods in bold print.

If you are following the carbohydrate-restricted version, don't eat the foods that are marked with an asterisk (*). You should eat larger quantities of no-carb foods than this food diary specifies.

"To love and be loved is to
feel the sun from both sides."

—David Viscott

Goals for Thursday:

Physical: _____
_____
_____

Mental: _____
_____
_____

Spiritual: _____
_____
_____

Do I like myself? Do I love myself? _____
_____
_____
_____
_____
_____
_____
_____

What am I thankful for today? _____
_____
_____

One nice thing I've done for myself today... _____
_____
_____
_____

Day: Thursday

		Carbs	Calories
Meal 1	1 egg	0	75
	3 sausage links	0	200
	1 slice whole wheat bread	12	70
	4 slices bacon	**0**	**120**
	1/2 slice whole wheat bread	**6**	**35**
	1 tablespoon mayonnaise	**0**	**100**
	***1 tomato, sliced**	**6**	**30**
Meal 2	2 Keebler Harvest Bakery Multigrain crackers	11	70
	2 tablespoons vegetable cream cheese	2	90
	1/2 cup 1% fat cottage cheese	**5**	**80**
	1/2 cup baby carrots	**5**	**24**
Meal 3	Stir Fry of:		
	1 tablespoon olive oil	0	120
	6 ounces chicken breast	0	186
	1/2 cup onions	FREE	FREE
	1 cup mushrooms	FREE	FREE
	1 cup asparagus	FREE	FREE
	Curves shake with 8 oz. skim milk	**FREE**	**FREE**
Meal 4	Curves shake with 8 oz. skim milk	FREE	FREE
	3 ounces water-packed tuna	**0**	**90**
	Free Foods Salad		
	Salad Dressing (your choice)		
Meal 5	Beef Tenderloin with Blue Cheese (page 67)	1	383
	Free Foods Salad		
	Salad Dressing (your choice)		
	Stir Fry of:		
	1 tablespoon olive oil	**0**	**120**
	8 ounces chicken breast	**0**	**248**
	1/2 cup onion	**FREE**	**FREE**
	1/2 cup mushrooms	**FREE**	**FREE**
	1/2 cup asparagus	**FREE**	**FREE**
Meal 6	1 banana	26	106
	2 ounces cheddar cheese	0	220
	2 ounces Havarti cheese	**0**	**240**
	***1 medium orange**	**16**	**65**

Water: ☐☐☐☐☐☐☐

Vitamins: ☐☐☐

Totals for Day

Today's Exercise:

Curves Workout ♡

or

Aerobic ♡

_____

_____

Strength Training ♡

_____

_____

Stretching ♡

_____

_____

PHASE II - 1

If you are doing the 2nd week of Phase I, you need to eat the foods in bold print.

If you are following the carbohydrate-restricted version, don't eat the foods that are marked with an asterisk (*). You should eat larger quantities of no-carb foods than this food diary specifies.

105

"You need the serenity to accept the things you cannot change, the courage to change the things you can and the wisdom to know the difference."

—Reinhold Niebuhr

Goals for Friday:

Physical: _____
_____
_____

Mental: _____
_____
_____

Spiritual: _____
_____
_____

How do I feel about changes in my life? _____
_____
_____
_____
_____
_____

What am I thankful for today? _____
_____
_____

One nice thing I've done for myself today... _____
_____
_____
_____

Day: Friday

			Carbs	Calories
Meal 1		4 ounces plain yogurt	9	75
		1 cup strawberries	12	46
		3 ounces lean ham	**0**	**100**
		2 eggs	**0**	**150**
		*1/2 grapefruit	**12**	**46**
Meal 2		Curves shake with 8 oz. skim milk	FREE	FREE
		1/2 cup 1% fat cottage cheese	**5**	**80**
		1/2 cup cubed cantaloupe	**6**	**25**
Meal 3		8 ounces pork chop, lean, broiled	0	300
		1 cup zucchini, sautéed in:	FREE	FREE
		1 tablespoon olive oil	0	120
		8 ounces broiled salmon	**0**	**414**
		1 cup brussels sprouts	**FREE**	**FREE**
		1 tablespoon butter	**0**	**102**
Meal 4		2 ounces Cheddar cheese	0	220
		2 ounces lean ham	0	67
		2 ounces pistachio nuts, in shells	7	170
		Curves shake with 8 oz. skim milk	**FREE**	**FREE**
Meal 5		1 serving Beef and Vegetable Stew (page 66)	8	256
		Free Foods Salad		
		Salad Dressing (your choice)		
		Free Foods Salad		
		2 tablespoons shredded Parmesan cheese	**0**	**55**
		Salad Dressing (your choice)		
Meal 6		2 Keebler Harvest Bakery Multigrain crackers	11	70
		2 tablespoons peanut butter	7	190
		1 stalk celery	**FREE**	**FREE**
		1 tablespoon peanut butter	**4**	**95**
		*2 Keebler Harvest Bakery Multigrain crackers	**11**	**70**

Water: ☐☐☐☐☐☐☐☐   Totals for Day

Vitamins: ⬭ ⬭ ⬭

Today's Exercise:

Curves Workout ♡

or

Aerobic ♡

_____

_____

Strength Training ♡

_____

_____

Stretching ♡

_____

_____

PHASE II - 1

If you are doing the 2nd week of Phase I, you need to eat the foods in bold print.

If you are following the carbohydrate-restricted version, don't eat the foods that are marked with an asterisk (*). You should eat larger quantities of no-carb foods than this food diary specifies.

And do not set your heart on what you will eat or drink; do not worry about it.

Luke 12:29

Goals for Saturday:

Physical: _____

_____

_____

Mental: _____

_____

_____

Spiritual: _____

_____

_____

Do I live to eat or eat to live? _____

_____

_____

_____

_____

_____

_____

What am I thankful for today? _____

_____

_____

One nice thing I've done for myself today... _____

_____

_____

_____

_____

Day: Saturday

		Carbs	Calories
Meal 1	1 slice whole wheat bread	12	70
	1 ounce Havarti cheese	0	120
	3 sausage links	0	200
	1/2 slice whole wheat bread	**6**	**35**
	1 ounce Havarti cheese	**0**	**120**
	3 sausage links	**0**	**200**
Meal 2	Curves shake with 8 oz. skim milk	FREE	FREE
	Curves shake with 8 oz. skim milk	**FREE**	**FREE**
Meal 3	6 ounces 93% lean ground beef, broiled	0	240
	1 ounce Cheddar cheese	0	110
	1/2 cup refried beans	25	120
	2 tablespoons salsa	2	10
	Free Foods Salad		
	Salad Dressing (your choice)		
Meal 4	1 ounce roasted and salted almonds	4	180
	6 ounces 93% hamburger, broiled	**0**	**240**
	***8 ounces V-8 juice**	**10**	**46**
Meal 5	1 serving Tofu Stir Fry (recipe page 72)	2	340
	8 ounces shrimp, broiled	**0**	**240**
	1 serving French Onion Soup (page 65)	**3**	**145**
	1/2 cup broccoli, steamed	**FREE**	**FREE**
	1 teaspoon butter	**0**	**34**
Meal 6	2 Turkey-Lettuce Wraps (recipe page 59)	4	152
	1 peach	9	37
	4 ounces plain yogurt	**9**	**75**
	***1/2 cup strawberries**	**6**	**23**

Water: ⬜⬜⬜⬜⬜⬜⬜⬜

Vitamins: ⬭⬭⬭

Totals for Day

Today's Exercise:

Curves Workout ♡

or

Aerobic ♡

_____

_____

Strength Training ♡

_____

_____

Stretching ♡

_____

_____

If you are doing the 2nd week of Phase I, you need to eat the foods in bold print.

If you are following the carbohydrate-restricted version, don't eat the foods that are marked with an asterisk (*). You should eat larger quantities of no-carb foods than this food diary specifies.

*"Come to me, all you who are weary
and burdened, and I will give you rest.*

Matthew 11:28

Goals for Sunday:

Physical: _____
_____
_____

Mental: _____
_____
_____

Spiritual: _____
_____
_____

Do I feel like I get enough sleep at night? How many hours
do I sleep on average? _____
_____
_____
_____
_____
_____
_____

What am I thankful for today? _____
_____
_____

One nice thing I've done for myself today... _____
_____
_____
_____
_____

Day: Sunday

		Carbs	Calories
Meal 1	2 eggs	0	150
	4 slices bacon	0	120
	4 ounces V-8 juice	5	23
	2 eggs	**0**	**150**
	3 sausage links	**0**	**200**
	***1/2 grapefruit**	**12**	**46**
Meal 2	Curves shake with 8 oz. skim milk	FREE	FREE
	4 ounces chicken breast, broiled	**0**	**124**
	1/2 cup green beans	**4**	**20**
	1 teaspoon butter	**0**	**34**
Meal 3	8 ounces chicken breast, broiled	0	248
	1 cup green beans	8	40
	1/2 tablespoon butter	0	51
	Free Foods Salad		
	Salad Dressing (your choice)		
	Free Foods Salad		
	Salad Dressing (your choice)		
Meal 4	1 serving Spicy Zucchini Boats (2 pieces) (recipe page 58)	2	195
	1/2 cup 1% fat cottage cheese	**5**	**80**
	1/2 cup cubed cantaloupe	**6**	**25**
	***2 Keebler Harvest Bakery Multigrain crackers**	**11**	**70**
Meal 5	8 ounces shrimp, broiled	0	240
	2 cups steamed spinach	FREE	FREE
	1 tablespoon butter	0	102
	1 medium orange	16	65
	8 ounces orange roughy sautéed in:	**0**	**216**
	1 tablespoon olive oil	**0**	**120**
	1 cup steamed cauliflower	**FREE**	**FREE**
	1/2 tablespoon butter	**0**	**51**
Meal 6	1/2 cup 1% fat cottage cheese	5	80
	1/2 cup cubed cantaloupe	6	25
	1 ounce cashews	7	170
	Curves shake with 8 oz. skim milk	**FREE**	**FREE**

Water: 🥛🥛🥛🥛🥛🥛🥛🥛

Vitamins: ⬭⬭⬭

Totals for Day

Today's Exercise:

Curves Workout ♡

or

Aerobic ♡

_____
_____

Strength Training ♡

_____
_____

Stretching ♡

_____
_____

If you are doing the 2nd week of Phase I, you need to eat the foods in bold print.

If you are following the carbohydrate-restricted version, don't eat the foods that are marked with an asterisk (*). You should eat larger quantities of no carb foods than this food diary specifies.

SHOPPING LIST–PHASE II, WEEK 2

Vegetables

____ $^1/_2$ cup asparagus
____ 1 cup broccoli florets
____ 1 cup brussels sprouts
____ 1 cup carrots
____ 1 cup cauliflower florets
____ 1 cup green beans
____ $^1/_2$ cup green peas
____ $^1/_2$ cups mushrooms, sliced
____ $^1/_2$ cup onion
____ 1 cup zucchini, sliced

Free Foods

____ enough for 5 salads

Dairy

____ 4 tablespoons butter
____ 5 ounces Cheddar cheese
____ $1^1/_2$ cups cottage cheese, lowfat (1%), small curd
____ 6 eggs
____ 5 ounces Havarti cheese
____ $^1/_2$ gallon milk, skim
____ 2 tablespoons Parmesan cheese, shredded
____ 2 tablespoons vegetable cream cheese
____ 8 ounces yogurt, plain, lowfat

Fruit

____ 1 small apple
____ $^1/_2$ banana
____ $^1/_4$ cup blueberries
____ 1 cup cantaloupe, cubed
____ $^1/_2$ cup seedless grapes
____ 1 cup strawberries
____ 1 cup watermelon, cubed

Meat

____ 24 ounces chicken breast (divided)
____ 16 ounces ground beef, 93% lean (divided)

____ 10 ounces ham, lean
____ 4 slices bacon
____ 6 breakfast sausage links
____ 6 ounces light smoked sausage
____ 16 ounces shrimp
____ 8 ounces orange roughy

Starches

____ 4 Keebler Harvest Bakery Multigrain crackers
____ 2 pieces Holland Rusk Dry Toast
____ 4 Rye Krisp crackers
____ 1 slice whole wheat bread

Other

____ 2 ounces roasted and salted cashews
____ 2 ounces pistachio nuts, in shells
____ 2 tablespoons peanut butter
____ $^1/_2$ cup refried beans
____ 4 ounces rosé wine
____ $^1/_2$ cup sauerkraut
____ 2 tablespoons salsa
____ 24 ounces V-8 juice
____ $^1/_2$ cup French vanilla ice cream

Recipes this week

____ Beef Tenderloin with Blue Cheese, page 67
____ Easy Frittata, page 68
____ French Onion Soup, page 65
____ Greek Salad, page 63
____ Italian Stuffed Mushrooms, page 60
____ Parmesan Vegetable Stir-Fry, page 73
____ Sherry-Mushroom Chicken, page 70
____ Spinach Salad, page 62
____ Tofu Stir-Fry, page 72
____ Tuna Salad, page 61

PHASE II
~ WEEK 2 ~

You should expect to lose 1-2 pounds per week during Phase II.
Your weight loss will begin to slow as your metabolism decreases.
Losing a pound or more of body fat weekly is worth the effort.
If you are following the higher protein method and your weight loss drops below
1 pound per week during Phase II, you should switch to the calorie-restricted version.

~

HIGHER PROTEIN/LOW CARBOHYDRATE

For the higher protein/low carbohydrate version, you should:

Enjoy unlimited amounts of lean meats, cheeses, eggs, seafood and poultry
(baked, broiled, or boiled—never fried).

Eat moderate to lower amounts of fat.
Limit your carbohydrate intake to 40-60 grams per day
(not counting free foods).

Eat, but don't cheat!

CALORIE-RESTRICTED

For the calorie-restricted version, you should:

Eat no more than 1600 calories per day
(not counting free foods).

Consume 40% of those calories in the form of protein foods.

Consume no more than 60 grams of carbohydrates per day
(not counting free foods).

~

HINT: You are not required to eat the meals in the order they are listed.
Feel free to adjust them to your lifestyle and schedule.

EXERCISE HELPS

List the five components of a balanced workout:

1. _____
2. _____
3. _____
4. _____
5. _____

What are your three favorite types of exercise?

1. _____
   _____
2. _____
   _____
3. _____
   _____

Why do you like them?

_____
_____
_____
_____

Strength training protects muscle mass, even while we are losing weight. Women sometimes avoid strength training because they do not want to develop huge muscles. The strength training component of the Curves Workout will not encourage the development of bulky muscles.

Aerobic exercise (cardio) is a vital part of our fitness plan. It conditions your body to better utilize body fat. If your goal is to attain a moderate level of fitness and encourage weight loss, you do not need to raise your heart rate above 60% to 70% of its maximum capacity.

Another part of our plan is stretching, which helps prevent soreness after a workout and can also help to prevent injuries. Always stretch after your workout.

Along with warming up and cooling down, strength training, cardio, and stretching make up a complete workout.

PHASE II - 2

DON'T QUIT

It is too easy to confuse disappointment with disaster. Maybe you haven't done a very good job of sticking to the 6 week challenge plan so far. Maybe you have only made it to Curves one time and haven't done any other form of exercise. Maybe you fell off the wagon just last week by going out to dinner and eating lots of bread and pasta. Every day is a new day and every meal is a chance to regain your good habits. Don't let your lack of perfection give you an excuse to quit.

Maybe other people are getting more results than you are. Don't let it get you down. You can only be responsible for your own body. Choose to be inspired by the good things happening to others—don't be jealous or mad.

All any of us can do is the best we can do, every day. So choose to do your best and don't give up. Remember that two steps forward and one step back will still get you there.

List 3 reasons you have been tempted to quit this 6-week challenge:
1._____
2._____
3._____

List 3 reasons to stick with it:
1._____
2._____
3._____

Describe your worst failure in following the plan so far:
_____
_____
_____
_____

Bear with each other and forgive whatever
grievances you may have against one another.
Forgive as the Lord forgave you.

Colossians 3:13

Goals for Monday:

Physical: _____

_____

_____

Mental: _____

_____

_____

Spiritual: _____

_____

_____

Is there any relationship in my life that needs forgiveness and healing? _____

_____

_____

_____

_____

_____

_____

What am I thankful for today? _____

_____

_____

One nice thing I've done for myself today... _____

_____

_____

Day: Monday

			Carbs	Calories
Meal 1		½ cup 1% fat cottage cheese	5	80
		½ cup seedless grapes	14	57
Meal 2		Curves shake with 8 oz. skim milk	FREE	FREE
Meal 3		8 ounces 93% lean ground beef, broiled	0	320
		1 cup cooked carrots	11	48
		½ tablespoon butter	0	51
		Free Foods Salad		
		Salad Dressing (your choice)		
Meal 4		⅔ cup tuna salad (recipe page 61)	3	258
		2 Rye Krisp crackers	11	60
Meal 5		8 ounces chicken breast, broiled	0	248
		Parmesan Vegetable Stir Fry (recipe page 73)	0	175
		8 ounces V-8 juice	10	46
Meal 6		2 ounces lean ham	0	67
		1 ounce Havarti cheese	0	120

Water: ▢ ▢ ▢ ▢ ▢ ▢ ▢

Vitamins: ▢ ▢ ▢

Totals for Day

Today's Exercise:

Curves Workout ♡

or

Aerobic ♡

_____

_____

Strength Training ♡

_____

_____

Stretching ♡

_____

_____

Today you need to go to Curves to be weighed and have your body fat tested. Record your results here:

Weight_____

% Body Fat _____

Pounds of
Body Fat _____

Also record your results on the chart on page 26.

TIP:
The ingredients for the recipes are not included in your shopping list—plan ahead so you are prepared.

PHASE II - 2

"Everyone wants to live on top of the mountain, but all the happiness and growth occurs from climbing it."

—Author unknown

Goals for Tuesday:

Physical: _____

_____

_____

Mental: _____

_____

_____

Spiritual: _____

_____

_____

When was the last time I had fun with others? _____

_____

_____

_____

_____

_____

_____

_____

What am I thankful for today? _____

_____

_____

One nice thing I've done for myself today... _____

_____

_____

_____

_____

PHASE II - 2

Day: Tuesday

		Carbs	Calories
Meal 1	2 eggs	0	150
	3 ounces lean ham	0	100
	1/2 tablespoon butter	0	51
	1 piece Holland Rusk Dry Toast	6	30
Meal 2	1/2 cup cubed cantaloupe	6	25
	1/2 cup 1% fat cottage cheese	5	80
	1 ounce roasted and salted cashews	7	170
Meal 3	1 serving Greek Salad (recipe page 63)	6	348
Meal 4	Curves shake with 8 oz. skim milk	FREE	FREE
Meal 5	8 ounces broiled orange roughy	0	216
	1 cup steamed cauliflower	FREE	FREE
	1/2 tablespoon butter	0	51
	1 serving French Onion Soup (recipe page 65)	3	145
Meal 6	1 ounce Havarti cheese	0	120
	1 small apple	20	80

Water: ⊔ ⊔ ⊔ ⊔ ⊔ ⊔ ⊔ ⊔

Vitamins: ⬭ ⬭ ⬭

Totals for Day

Today's Exercise:

Curves Workout ♡

or

Aerobic ♡

_____

_____

Strength Training ♡

_____

_____

Stretching ♡

_____

_____

*"I thought in my heart, 'Come now, I will test you
with pleasure to find out what is good.'
But that also proved to be meaningless."*

Ecclesiastes 2:1

Goals for Wednesday:

Physical: _____

_____

_____

Mental: _____

_____

_____

Spiritual: _____

_____

_____

What bores me? _____

_____

_____

_____

_____

_____

What am I thankful for today? _____

_____

_____

One nice thing I've done for myself today... _____

_____

_____

_____

Day: Wednesday

		Carbs	Calories
Meal 1	4 ounces plain yogurt	9	75
	1/4 cup blueberries	7	27
Meal 2	Curves shake with 8 oz. skim milk	FREE	FREE
Meal 3	1 serving Spinach Salad (recipe page 62)		
	with 2 tablespoons Orange Vinaigrette	3	101
	8 ounces chicken breast, broiled	0	248
Meal 4	2 tablespoons peanut butter	7	190
	2 Rye Krisp Crackers	11	60
	8 ounces V-8 juice	10	46
Meal 5	6 ounces light smoked sausage	12	330
	1/2 cup sauerkraut	FREE	FREE
	1 cup zucchini sautéed in:	FREE	FREE
	1 tablespoon olive oil	0	120
Meal 6	3 ounces lean ham	0	100
	2 ounces Havarti cheese	0	240

Water: 🥛🥛🥛🥛🥛🥛🥛   Totals for Day

Vitamins: ⬭ ⬭ ⬭

Curves Workout ♡

or

Aerobic ♡

_____

_____

Strength Training ♡

_____

_____

Stretching ♡

_____

_____

PHASE II - 2

TIP:
Plain lowfat yogurt and 1% cottage cheese are interchangeable in equal amounts.

121

"Twenty years from now you will be more disappointed by the things that you didn't do than by the ones you did do. So throw off the bowlines. Sail away from the safe harbor. Catch the trade winds in your sails. Explore. Dream. Discover."

—Mark Twain

Goals for Thursday:

Physical: _____

_____

_____

Mental: _____

_____

_____

Spiritual: _____

_____

_____

What never bores me? _____

_____

_____

_____

_____

_____

What am I thankful for today? _____

_____

_____

One nice thing I've done for myself today... _____

_____

_____

Day: Thursday

		Carbs	Calories
Meal 1	1 egg	0	75
	3 sausage links	0	200
	1 piece Holland Rusk Dry Toast	6	30
Meal 2	2 Keebler Harvest Bakery Multigrain crackers	11	70
	2 tablespoons vegetable cream cheese	2	90
Meal 3	1 serving Sherry-Mushroom Chicken (page 70)	3	288
	1/2 cup steamed asparagus	FREE	FREE
	1 teaspoon butter	0	34
	Free Foods Salad		
	Salad Dressing (your choice)		
Meal 4	Curves shake with 8 oz. skim milk	FREE	FREE
Meal 5	Stir Fry of:		
	1 tablespoon olive oil	0	120
	8 ounces shrimp	0	240
	1/2 cup onions	FREE	FREE
	1/2 cup mushrooms	FREE	FREE
	1/2 cup green peas	11	60
Meal 6	1 ounce roasted and salted cashews	7	170
	1 cup cubed watermelon	12	50
	1 ounce cheddar cheese	0	110

Water: ▯▯▯▯▯▯▯▯   Totals for Day

Vitamins: ⬭ ⬭ ⬭

Today's Exercise:

Curves Workout ♡

or

Aerobic ♡

_____

_____

Strength Training ♡

_____

_____

Stretching ♡

_____

_____

PHASE II - 2

"Habit is either the best of servants
or the worst of masters."

—Nathaniel Emmons

Goals for Friday:

Physical: _____
_____
_____

Mental: _____
_____
_____

Spiritual: _____
_____
_____

How important is food to you? Do you think of it very often?
Do you feel disciplined in your management of food?

_____
_____
_____
_____
_____
_____
_____
_____

What am I thankful for today? _____
_____
_____

One nice thing I've done for myself today... _____
_____
_____

Day: Friday

			Carbs	Calories
Meal 1		4 ounces plain yogurt	9	75
		1 cup strawberries	12	46
		2 ounces pistachio nuts, in shells	7	170
Meal 2		Curves shake with 8 oz. skim milk	FREE	FREE
Meal 3		1 serving Easy Frittata (recipe page 68)	4	325
		Free Foods Salad		
		Salad Dressing (your choice)		
Meal 4		1 serving Italian Stuffed Mushrooms (recipe page 60)	6	145
Meal 5		1 serving Beef Tenderloin with Blue Cheese (recipe page 67)	1	383
		1 cup brussels sprouts	FREE	FREE
		1/2 tablespoon butter	0	51
Meal 6		2 ounces lean ham	0	67
		2 Keebler Harvest Bakery Multigrain crackers	11	70
		2 ounces Cheddar cheese	0	220

Water: ▯▯▯▯▯▯▯   Totals for Day
Vitamins: ⬭ ⬭ ⬭

Today's Exercise:

Curves Workout ♡

or

Aerobic ♡

_____
_____

Strength Training ♡

_____
_____

Stretching ♡

_____

PHASE II - 2

TIP:
Check labels on ham. Some ham has a sugar cured flavoring added, which adds carbs.

Therefore do not worry about tomorrow,
for tomorrow will worry about itself.
Each day has enough trouble of its own.

Matthew 6:34

Goals for Saturday:

Physical: _____
_____
_____

Mental: _____
_____
_____

Spiritual: _____
_____
_____

What am I worried or concerned about today? _____
_____
_____
_____
_____
_____

What am I thankful for today? _____
_____
_____

One nice thing I've done for myself today... _____
_____
_____
_____
_____

Day: Saturday

		Carbs	Calories
Meal 1	1 slice whole wheat bread	12	70
	1 ounce Havarti cheese	0	120
	3 sausage links	0	200
Meal 2	Curves shake with 8 oz. skim milk	FREE	FREE
Meal 3	8 ounces 93% lean ground beef, broiled	0	320
	2 ounces Cheddar cheese	0	220
	1/2 cup refried beans	25	120
	2 tablespoons salsa	2	10
Meal 4	1/2 banana	13	53
Meal 5	1 hard boiled egg	0	75
	Free Foods Salad		
	Salad Dressing (your choice)		
Meal 6	1 serving Tofu Stir Fry (recipe page 72)	2	340

Water: 🥛🥛🥛🥛🥛🥛🥛🥛
Vitamins: ⬭ ⬭ ⬭

Totals for Day

PHASE II - 2

127

"The Hunger for Love is much more difficult
to remove than the Hunger for Bread"
—*Mother Teresa*

Goals for Sunday:

Physical: _____

_____

_____

Mental: _____

_____

_____

Spiritual: _____

_____

_____

Am I trying to fill a void in my life by eating? by exercising?
by dieting? _____

_____

_____

_____

_____

What am I thankful for today? _____

_____

_____

One nice thing I've done for myself today... _____

_____

_____

_____

Reminder - Go to Curves Monday to be measured and have
your weight and body fat tested. Record your results in the
charts on page 25 and 26.

Day: Sunday

		Carbs	Calories
Meal 1	2 eggs	0	150
	4 slices bacon	0	120
	8 ounces V-8 juice	10	46
Meal 2	¹/₂ cup 1% fat cottage cheese	5	80
	¹/₂ cup cubed cantaloupe	6	25
Meal 3	8 ounces chicken breast, broiled	0	248
	1 cup green beans	8	40
	¹/₂ tablespoon butter	0	51
	2 tablespoons shredded Parmesan cheese	0	55
	Free Foods Salad		
	Salad Dressing (your choice)		
Meal 4	¹/₂ cup French vanilla ice cream	15	160
	4 ounce glass of rosé wine	6	100
Meal 5	8 ounces shrimp sautéed in:	0	240
	1 tablespoon olive oil	0	120
	1 cup steamed broccoli	FREE	FREE
	1 tablespoon butter	0	102
Meal 6	Curves shake with 8 oz. skim milk	FREE	FREE

Water: 🥛🥛🥛🥛🥛🥛🥛🥛

Vitamins: 💊💊💊

Totals for Day		

Today's Exercise:

Curves Workout ♡

or

Aerobic ♡

_____

_____

Strength Training ♡

_____

_____

Stretching ♡

_____

_____

PHASE II - 2

SHOPPING LIST–PHASE II, WEEK 3

Vegetables
- ____1 cup asparagus
- ____1 cup broccoli florets
- ____1 cup carrots
- ____2 cups snow peas
- ____2 cups spinach, fresh
- ____1 cup zucchini, sliced

_____

Free Foods
- ____enough for 6 salads

Dairy
- ____3 tablespoons butter
- ____4 ounces Cheddar cheese
- ____2 cups cottage cheese, lowfat (1%), small curd
- ____6 eggs
- ____7 ounces Havarti cheese
- ____1/2 gallon milk, skim
- ____2 ounces Monterey Jack cheese
- ____2 tablespoons vegetable cream cheese
- ____4 ounces yogurt, plain, lowfat

Fruit
- ____1 small apple
- ____1/2 cup blueberries
- ____1 1/2 cups cantaloupe, cubed
- ____1 medium orange
- ____1 cup strawberries
- ____1 cup watermelon, cubed

_____

Meat and Seafood
- ____16 ounces chicken breast (divided)
- ____14 ounces ground beef, 93% lean (divided)
- ____8 ounces sirloin steak
- ____4 ounces deli roast beef
- ____3 ounces ham, lean
- ____9 breakfast sausage links
- ____4 slices bacon
- ____6 ounces salmon
- ____8 ounces shrimp
- ____8 ounces orange roughy
- ____6 ounces light smoked sausage

_____

Starches
- ____1 piece Holland Rusk Dry Toast
- ____2 Keebler Harvest Bakery Multigrain crackers
- ____4 Rye Krisp crackers
- ____3 slices whole wheat bread

_____

Other
- ____1 tablespoon barbeque sauce
- ____1 tablespoon mayonnaise
- ____3 ounces roasted and salted cashews
- ____1 ounce roasted and salted almonds
- ____2 tablespoons peanut butter
- ____1/2 cup French vanilla ice cream
- ____1/2 cup refried beans
- ____2 tablespoons salsa
- ____1/2 cup sauerkraut
- ____8 ounces V-8 juice
- ____4 ounces rosé wine

_____

Recipes this week
- ____Beef and Vegetable Stew, page 66
- ____Creamy Coleslaw, page 64
- ____Easy Frittata, page 68
- ____Greek Salad, page 63
- ____Parmesan Vegetable Stir-Fry, page 73
- ____Sherry-Mushroom Chicken, page 70
- ____Tuna Salad, page 61
- ____Turkey-Lettuce Wraps, page 59

PHASE II

~ WEEK 3 ~

As long as you are losing at least 1 pound per week you should continue on Phase II.
If your weight loss drops below 1 pound per week during Phase II,
even after switching to the calorie-restricted version,
you should move to Phase III because you have hit a plateau.

~

HIGHER PROTEIN/LOW CARBOHYDRATE

For the higher protein/low carbohydrate version, you should:

Enjoy unlimited amounts of lean meats, cheeses, eggs, seafood and poultry
(baked, broiled, or boiled—never fried).

Eat moderate to lower amounts of fat.
Limit your carbohydrate intake to 40-60 grams per day
(not counting free foods).

Eat, but don't cheat!

CALORIE-RESTRICTED

For the calorie-restricted version, you should:

Eat no more than 1600 calories per day
(not counting free foods).

Consume 40% of those calories in the form of protein foods.

Consume no more than 60 grams of carbohydrates per day
(not counting free foods).

~

HINT: You are not required to eat the meals in the order they are listed.
Feel free to adjust them to your lifestyle and schedule.

SELF LABELS & SELF TALK

List 6 of your good qualities:
1. _____
2. _____
3. _____
4. _____
5. _____
6. _____

List 3 nice names for yourself:
1. _____
2. _____
3. _____

Write a daily affirmation for yourself:

_____
_____
_____
_____
_____
_____

Children get stuck with labels and nicknames that may or may not have any basis in truth. Perhaps your childhood nickname was "trouble." Are you still "trouble?" Maybe you were "Mommy's good girl." Does that feel like a burden now?

As adults, we are free to create our own self labels. It is good to work on thinking of yourself in complimentary terms. People who care about you are already referring to you by nice names.

Self talk is going on in your head all day long. So take the opportunity to say nice things to yourself. Congratulate yourself for doing your best on this 6-week challenge. Praise yourself for learning to enjoy different foods. Acknowledge your right to put your needs ahead of the needs of others for a while.

PHASE II - 3

HABITS

It takes about 30 days to acquire a habit—good or bad. At this point in the 6 week challenge, you should be acquiring some new habits. The day to day part of following the plan should be getting easier, because it should be becoming routine. If you are trying to drop a lot of bad habits during this 6 week challenge, you may be struggling. Keep doing the best you can every day. Now is not the time to give up. You have just two more weeks to complete the challenge.

Perhaps some of your customs are getting in the way of following the plan. For instance, if you are a late night snacker, maybe you could go to bed sooner. If you like to eat popcorn with your family while you watch TV, could you eat celery or a small amount of nuts instead? Could you watch less TV? Could you keep your hands busy with needlework or knitting?

Try to make your habits work to your advantage.

List 3 habits that are making it difficult for you to follow the plan:
1._____
2._____
3._____

List 3 things you can do to circumvent those habits:
1._____
2._____
3._____

List 3 good new habits you have gained so far:
1._____
2._____
3._____

Do not judge, and you will not be judged.
Do not condemn, and you will not be condemned.
Forgive, and you will be forgiven.

Luke 6:37

Goals for Monday:

Physical: _____

_____

_____

Mental: _____

_____

_____

Spiritual: _____

_____

_____

Is there anyone I am unwilling to forgive? Is there anyone I do
not want to talk to? _____

_____

_____

_____

_____

_____

_____

What am I thankful for today? _____

_____

_____

One nice thing I've done for myself today... _____

_____

_____

Day: Monday

		Carbs	Calories
Meal 1	1/2 cup 1% fat cottage cheese	5	80
	1 cup strawberries	12	46
Meal 2	Curves shake with 8 oz. skim milk	FREE	FREE
Meal 3	8 ounces 93% lean ground beef, broiled	0	320
	1 cup cooked carrots	11	48
	1 teaspoon butter	0	34
	Free Foods Salad		
	Salad Dressing (your choice)		
Meal 4	2/3 cup tuna salad (recipe page 61)	3	258
	2 Rye Krisp crackers	11	60
Meal 5	8 ounces chicken breast, broiled	0	248
	1 tablespoon barbeque sauce	6	25
	1 serving Creamy Coleslaw (recipe page 64)	3	78
	1 cup steamed broccoli	FREE	FREE
	1 tablespoon butter	0	102
Meal 6	2 ounces Havarti cheese	0	240

Water: ⌴ ⌴ ⌴ ⌴ ⌴ ⌴ ⌴

Vitamins: ⌵ ⌵ ⌵

Totals for Day

Today's Exercise:

Curves Workout ♡

or

Aerobic ♡

_____

_____

Strength Training ♡

_____

_____

Stretching ♡

_____

_____

Today you need to go to Curves to be weighed and have your body fat tested. Record your results here:

Weight_____

% Body Fat _____

Pounds of
Body Fat _____

Record your results on the chart on page 26. You also need to have measurements taken and recorded in the chart on page 25 (Week 4 Measurements)

PHASE II - 3

TIP:
Don't forget to stretch after your workout — your body will thank you!

135

"When you have a dream
you've got to grab it and never let go."

—*Carol Burnett*

Goals for Tuesday:

Physical: _____

_____

_____

Mental: _____

_____

_____

Spiritual: _____

_____

_____

If I had unlimited money and time, and could do anything in
the world, what would it be?_____

_____

_____

_____

_____

_____

What am I thankful for today? _____

_____

_____

One nice thing I've done for myself today... _____

_____

_____

_____

_____

Day: Tuesday

		Carbs	Calories
Meal 1	2 eggs	0	150
	3 ounces lean ham	0	100
Meal 2	1/2 cup 1% fat cottage cheese	5	80
	1 ounce roasted and salted cashews	7	170
Meal 3	1 serving Greek Salad (recipe page 63)	6	348
	1/2 cup French vanilla ice cream	15	160
Meal 4	Curves shake with 8 oz. skim milk	FREE	FREE
Meal 5	8 ounces broiled orange roughy	0	216
	1 cup snow peas	FREE	FREE
	1/2 tablespoon butter	0	51
Meal 6	2 ounces Monterey Jack cheese	0	220
	1 small apple	20	80

Water: ▯▯▯▯▯▯▯▯

Vitamins: ⬭ ⬭ ⬭

Totals for Day

Today's Exercise:

Curves Workout ♡

or

Aerobic ♡

_____

_____

Strength Training ♡

_____

_____

Stretching ♡

_____

_____

PHASE II - 3

137

"Each friend represents a world in us, a world possibly not born until they arrive, and it is only by this meeting that a new world is born."

—Anais Nin

Goals for Wednesday:

Physical: _____

_____

_____

Mental: _____

_____

_____

Spiritual: _____

_____

_____

What are 5 things I enjoyed doing with others in the last year? _____

_____

_____

_____

_____

_____

_____

What am I thankful for today? _____

_____

_____

One nice thing I've done for myself today... _____

_____

_____

PHASE II - 3

Day: Wednesday

		Carbs	Calories
Meal 1	4 ounces plain yogurt	9	75
	1/2 cup blueberries	14	54
Meal 2	Curves shake with 8 oz. skim milk	FREE	FREE
Meal 3	8 ounces sirloin steak, broiled	0	430
	Free Foods Salad		
	Salad Dressing (your choice)		
Meal 4	2 tablespoons peanut butter	7	190
	2 Rye Krisp Crackers	11	60
Meal 5	6 ounces light smoked sausage	12	330
	1/2 cup sauerkraut	FREE	FREE
	1 cup zucchini sautééd in:	FREE	FREE
	1 tablespoon olive oil	0	120
Meal 6	2 ounces Havarti cheese	0	240

Water: 🥛🥛🥛🥛🥛🥛🥛
Vitamins: ⬭ ⬭ ⬭

Totals for Day

Today's Exercise:

Curves Workout ♡

or

Aerobic ♡

_____
_____

Strength Training ♡

_____
_____

Stretching ♡

_____
_____

TIP:
Make sure you use a salad dressing you really enjoy. Have several on hand so you don't get bored.

Nobody should seek his own good,
but the good of others.

1 Corinthians 10:24

Goals for Thursday:

Physical: _____

_____

Mental: _____

_____

Spiritual: _____

_____

Who is the most important person in my life and why?

_____

_____

_____

_____

_____

_____

_____

What am I thankful for today? _____

_____

_____

One nice thing I've done for myself today... _____

_____

_____

_____

_____

Day: Thursday _____

		Carbs	Calories
Meal 1	1 egg	0	75
	3 sausage links	0	200
	1 piece Holland Rusk Dry Toast	6	30
Meal 2	2 Keebler Harvest Bakery Multigrain crackers	11	70
	2 tablespoons vegetable cream cheese	2	90
Meal 3	1 serving Sherry-Mushroom Chicken (page 70)	3	288
	1 cup steamed asparagus	FREE	FREE
	1/2 tablespoon butter	0	51
Meal 4	Curves shake with 8 oz. skim milk	FREE	FREE
Meal 5	1 serving Beef and Vegetable Stew (recipe page 66)	8	256
	Free Foods Salad		
	Salad Dressing (your choice)		
Meal 6	1 ounce roasted and salted cashews	7	170
	1 cup cubed watermelon	12	50
	2 ounces cheddar cheese	0	220

Water: 🥛🥛🥛🥛🥛🥛🥛
Vitamins: ⬭ ⬭ ⬭

Totals for Day	

Today's Exercise:

Curves Workout ♡

or

Aerobic ♡

_____

Strength Training ♡

_____

_____

Stretching ♡

_____

_____

PHASE II - 3

141

"Regret is an appalling waste of energy; you can't build on it; it is good only for wallowing."

—Katherine Mansfield

Goals for Friday:

Physical: _____

_____

Mental: _____

_____

Spiritual: _____

_____

What is the biggest regret in my life? Can I do anything to change it? _____

_____

_____

_____

_____

_____

_____

_____

What am I thankful for today? _____

_____

_____

One nice thing I've done for myself today... _____

_____

_____

_____

Day: Friday

		Carbs	Calories
Meal 1	2 eggs	0	150
	4 slices bacon	0	120
	1/2 cup cubed cantaloupe	6	25
Meal 2	Curves shake with 8 oz. skim milk	FREE	FREE
Meal 3	1 serving Easy Frittata (recipe page 68)	4	325
	Free Foods Salad		
	Salad Dressing (your choice)		
Meal 4	1 ounce Cheddar cheese	0	110
	4 ounces deli roast beef	4	120
	2 slices whole wheat bread	24	140
	1 tablespoon mayonnaise	0	100
Meal 5	1/2 cup 1% fat cottage cheese	5	80
	1 ounce roasted and salted almonds	4	180
Meal 6	2 Turkey-Lettuce Wraps (recipe page 59)	4	152

Water: ⬜⬜⬜⬜⬜⬜⬜⬜
Vitamins: ⬜⬜⬜

Totals for Day

Today's Exercise:

Curves Workout ♡

or

Aerobic ♡

_____
_____

Strength Training ♡

_____
_____

Stretching ♡

_____
_____

PHASE II - 3

TIP:
Don't eat only iceberg lettuce, try some other varieties. It will keep your salads interesting, and keep you eating them.

"The ultimate measure of a man is not where he stands in moments of comfort and convenience but where he stands at times of challenge and controversy."

— Martin Luther King

Goals for Saturday:

Physical: _____

_____

_____

Mental: _____

_____

_____

Spiritual: _____

_____

_____

If I could do anything in the world without fearing rejection, what would it be? _____

_____

_____

_____

_____

_____

What am I thankful for today? _____

_____

_____

One nice thing I've done for myself today... _____

_____

_____

Day: Saturday

			Carbs	Calories
Meal 1		1 slice whole wheat bread	12	70
		1 ounce Havarti cheese	0	120
		3 sausage links	0	200
Meal 2		Curves shake with 8 oz. skim milk	FREE	FREE
Meal 3		6 ounces 93% lean ground beef, broiled	0	240
		1 ounce Cheddar cheese	0	110
		1/2 cup refried beans	25	120
		2 tablespoons salsa	2	10
Meal 4		1 ounce roasted and salted cashews	7	170
Meal 5		6 ounces broiled salmon	0	311
		1 serving Parmesan Vegetable Stir Fry (recipe page 73)	0	175
Meal 6		Free Foods Salad		
		Salad Dressing (your choice)		

Water: ▯▯▯▯▯▯▯▯

Vitamins: ⬭ ⬭ ⬭

Totals for Day

Today's Exercise:

Curves Workout ♡

or

Aerobic ♡

_____

_____

Strength Training ♡

_____

_____

Stretching ♡

_____

_____

*"Nothing would be done at all if we
waited until we could do it so well that
no one could find fault with it."*

–Cardinal Newman

Goals for Sunday:

Physical: _____
_____
_____

Mental: _____
_____
_____

Spiritual: _____
_____
_____

Do I procrastinate? What am I avoiding?_____
_____
_____
_____
_____
_____
_____
_____

What am I thankful for today? _____
_____
_____

One nice thing I've done for myself today... _____
_____
_____
_____

Day: Sunday

		Carbs	Calories
Meal 1	1 egg	0	75
	3 sausage links	0	200
	8 ounces V-8 juice	10	46
Meal 2	¹/₂ cup 1% fat cottage cheese	5	80
	¹/₂ cup cubed cantaloupe	6	25
Meal 3	8 ounces chicken breast, broiled	0	248
	1 cup snow peas	FREE	FREE
	¹/₂ tablespoon butter	0	51
	1 medium orange	16	65
Meal 4	2 ounces Havarti cheese	0	240
	4 ounce glass of rosé wine	6	100
Meal 5	8 ounces shrimp sautéed in:	0	240
	1 tablespoon olive oil	0	120
	2 cups spinach	FREE	FREE
	Free Foods Salad		
	Salad Dressing (your choice)		
Meal 6	Curves shake with 8 oz. skim milk	FREE	FREE

Water: 🥛🥛🥛🥛🥛🥛🥛
Vitamins: ⬭ ⬭ ⬭

Totals for Day

Today's Exercise:

Curves Workout ♡

or

Aerobic ♡

_____

_____

Strength Training ♡

_____

_____

Stretching ♡

_____

_____

SHOPPING LIST–PHASE II, WEEK 4

Vegetables
____1 cup asparagus
____1 cup broccoli florets
____1 cup cauliflower florets
____1 cup green peas
____1 cup snow peas
____1 cup spinach, fresh
____1 cup zucchini, sliced

_____

Free Foods
____enough for 6 salads

Dairy
____4 tablespoons butter
____2 cups cottage cheese,
    lowfat (1%), small curd
____8 eggs
____7 ounces Cheddar cheese
____1 ounce Havarti cheese
____5 ounces Monterey Jack
    cheese
____1 ounce Swiss cheese
____ $1/2$ gallon milk, skim
____2 tablespoons vegetable
    cream cheese
____4 ounces yogurt, plain,
    lowfat

Fruit
____$1/2$ cup blueberries
____$1^1/2$ cups cantaloupe, cubed
____1 medium orange
____1 peach
____1 plum
____$1^1/2$ cups strawberries
____$1/2$ cup watermelon, cubed

_____

Meat
____10 ounces chicken breast
    (divided)
____8 ounce pork chop, lean
____14 ounces ground beef,
    93% lean (divided)
____4 ounces deli turkey breast

____4 ounces ham, lean (divided)
____9 breakfast sausage links
____4 slices bacon
____8 ounces orange roughy
____8 ounces salmon
____8 ounces shrimp

_____

Starches
____1 piece Holland Rusk
    Dry Toast
____4 Keebler Harvest Bakery
    Multigrain crackers
____6 Rye Krisp crackers
____4 slices whole wheat bread

Other
____2 ounces dry roasted peanuts
____2 ounces roasted and salted
    cashews
____$1/2$ cup refried beans
____2 tablespoons salsa
____8 ounces V-8 juice
____8 ounces rosé wine
____1 tablespoon mayonnaise

Recipes this week
____Beef and Vegetable Stew,
    page 66
____Beef Tenderloin with Blue
    Cheese, page 67
____Frozen Chocolate Mousse,
    page 74
____Greek Salad, page 63
____Italian Stuffed Mushrooms,
    page 60
____Jamaican Seafood Medley,
    page 71
____Spicy Chili Pork Chops,
    page 69
____Spicy Zucchini Boats,
    page 58
____Spinach Salad, page 62
____Turkey-Lettuce Wraps,
    page 59

PHASE II - 3

148

PHASE II
~ WEEK 4 ~

As long as you are losing at least 1 pound per week you should continue on Phase II.
If your weight loss drops below 1 pound per week during Phase II,
you should move to Phase III.

~

HIGHER PROTEIN/LOW CARBOHYDRATE

For the higher protein/low carbohydrate version, you should:

Enjoy unlimited amounts of lean meats, cheeses, eggs, seafood and poultry
(baked, broiled, or boiled—never fried).

Eat moderate to lower amounts of fat.
Limit your carbohydrate intake to 40-60 grams per day
(not counting free foods).

Eat, but don't cheat!

CALORIE-RESTRICTED

For the calorie-restricted version, you should:

Eat no more than 1600 calories per day
(not counting free foods).

Consume 40% of those calories in the form of protein foods.

Consume no more than 60 grams of carbohydrates per day
(not counting free foods).

~

HINT: You are not required to eat the meals in the order they are listed.
Feel free to adjust them to your lifestyle and schedule.

PHASE II - 4

NEEDS

List 5 foods you feel you cannot live without:

1. _____
2. _____
3. _____
4. _____
5. _____

List 3 foods that calm you down:

1. _____
2. _____
3. _____

List 3 foods that make you happy:

1. _____
2. _____
3. _____

Dr. Abraham Maslow created a model of our Hierarchy Of Needs, which describes how we prioritize. Our first priority is always our biological needs. This is good because it ensures the survival of our species. The next priority is for our safety, also vital to our survival. If both of these needs are being satisfied, then we may move on to our need for attachment to others. After that comes our need for esteem, and then our need to have a meaningful existence, also called self-actualization.

Our subconscious minds drive us to eat certain foods or quantities of food. Our food choices should meet our biological needs, and should not be driven by our subconscious. Our needs for security and self-esteem cannot really be taken care of by eating chocolate, and 5,000 calories every day will never satisfy our need to be loved.

PHASE II - 4

WANTS

Giving in to every desire is immature behavior, and will ultimately bring some bad consequence. It is important to be able to tell the difference between genuine needs (are you hungry?) and momentary wants (would you love to munch on a bag of potato chips?). Some women find that they must remove themselves from the presence of the desired food to keep from eating it. Don't feel silly if you have to do this—there is no shame in using your self control to avoid doing something you will regret later.

If cravings are a continual problem for you, maybe you need to examine the situations and people involved. You might start a cravings journal and take note of where you were, what time of the day it was, who was with you, and how you were feeling otherwise. This should not give you an excuse to overeat after every tense meeting, it should help to give you insight into your own thinking and help you to control yourself.

What are you craving right now?
_____
_____
_____

What will happen if you don't give in?
_____
_____
_____

What will happen if you do give in?
_____
_____
_____

Which consequence is more attractive to you?
_____

What will it take to let this craving pass by?
_____
_____

"Wonderful things start to happen when
you dream outside of your sleep."
—Richard Wilkins

Goals for Monday:

Physical: _____
_____
_____

Mental: _____
_____
_____

Spiritual: _____
_____
_____

What is the one dream for my life I am most eager to
achieve? _____
_____
_____
_____
_____
_____
_____

What am I thankful for today? _____
_____
_____

One nice thing I've done for myself today... _____
_____
_____
_____

Day: Monday

		Carbs	Calories
Meal 1	1/2 cup 1% fat cottage cheese	5	80
	1 cup strawberries	12	46
	2 Keebler Harvest Bakery Multigrain crackers	11	70
Meal 2	Curves shake with 8 oz. skim milk	FREE	FREE
Meal 3	8 ounces 93% lean ground beef, broiled	0	320
	1 cup zucchini, sauteed in:	FREE	FREE
	1 tablespoon olive oil	0	120
Meal 4	1 slice whole wheat bread	12	70
	4 ounces deli turkey breast	4	120
	1 ounce Swiss cheese	0	110
	1 tablespoon mayonnaise	0	100
Meal 5	1 serving Spicy Chili Pork Chops (recipe page 69)	4	219
	1 cup steamed cauliflower	FREE	FREE
	1/2 tablespoon butter	0	51
	Free Foods Salad		
	Salad Dressing (your choice)		
Meal 6	1 ounce Monterey Jack cheese	0	110
	4-ounce glass of rosé wine	6	100

Water: ⬚ ⬚ ⬚ ⬚ ⬚ ⬚ ⬚

Vitamins: ⬚ ⬚ ⬚

Totals for Day

Today's Exercise:

Curves Workout ♡

or

Aerobic ♡

_____

_____

Strength Training ♡

_____

_____

Stretching ♡

_____

_____

Today you need to go to Curves to be weighed and have your body fat tested. Record your results here:

Weight_____

% Body Fat _____

Pounds of Body Fat _____

Also record your results on the chart on page 26.

TIP:
Try some of the Curves shake variations (page 43) so you don't get bored.

PHASE II - 4

But when you pray, go into your room,
close the door and pray to your Father,
who is unseen. Then your Father, who sees
what is done in secret, will reward you.

Matthew 6:6

Goals for Tuesday:

Physical: _____
_____
_____

Mental: _____
_____
_____

Spiritual: _____
_____
_____

What are 5 things I enjoyed doing alone in the last year?
_____
_____
_____
_____
_____
_____

What am I thankful for today? _____
_____
_____

One nice thing I've done for myself today... _____
_____
_____
_____

Day: Tuesday

			Carbs	Calories
Meal 1		2 eggs	0	150
		4 slices bacon	0	120
		1 slice whole wheat bread	12	70
		1/2 tablespoon butter	0	51
Meal 2		1/2 cup cubed cantaloupe	6	25
		1/2 cup 1% fat cottage cheese	5	80
		2 Rye Krisp crackers	11	60
Meal 3		1 serving Greek Salad (recipe page 63)	6	348
Meal 4		Curves shake with 8 oz. skim milk	FREE	FREE
Meal 5		1 serving Jamaican Seafood Medley (recipe page 71)	6	283
Meal 6		2 ounces Cheddar cheese	0	220
		1 ounce roasted and salted cashews	7	170

Water: ⬭⬭⬭⬭⬭⬭⬭⬭
Vitamins: ⬭ ⬭ ⬭

Totals for Day

Today's Exercise:

Curves Workout ♡

or

Aerobic ♡

_____

_____

Strength Training ♡

_____

_____

Stretching ♡

_____

_____

PHASE II - 4

"He who accepts the unaltered philosophy of another is as ludicrous as he who dons his neighbor's hat, and infinitely more ridiculous."
— Paulette Goddard

Goals for Wednesday:

Physical: _____
_____
_____

Mental: _____
_____
_____

Spiritual: _____
_____
_____

What is my philosophy of life? _____
_____
_____
_____
_____
_____

What am I thankful for today? _____
_____
_____

One nice thing I've done for myself today... _____
_____
_____
_____
_____

Day: Wednesday

			Carbs	Calories
Meal 1		4 ounces plain yogurt	9	75
		1/2 cup blueberries	14	54
Meal 2		Curves shake with 8 oz. skim milk	FREE	FREE
Meal 3		8 ounce pork chop, broiled	0	300
		1 serving Spinach Salad (recipe page 62)		
		with 2 tablespoons Orange Vinaigrette	3	101
Meal 4		1 serving Italian Stuffed Mushrooms		
		(recipe page 60)	6	145
		8 ounces V-8 juice	10	46
Meal 5		1 serving Beef Tenderloin with Blue Cheese	1	383
		(recipe page 67)		
		1 cup green peas	11	60
		1/2 tablespoon butter	0	51
		Free Foods Salad		
		Salad Dressing (your choice)		
Meal 6		2 ounces lean ham	0	67
		2 ounces Monterey Jack cheese	0	220

Water: 🥛🥛🥛🥛🥛🥛🥛

Vitamins: 💊 💊 💊

Totals for Day

Today's Exercise:

Curves Workout ♡

or

Aerobic ♡

_____

_____

Strength Training ♡

_____

_____

Stretching ♡

_____

_____

TIP:
When someone says "it's too bad you can't eat this," reply "I could eat it, but I choose not to." Take responsibility for your choices.

PHASE II - 4

157

Each one should test his own actions.
Then he can take pride in himself without
comparing himself to somebody else, for
each one should carry his own load.

Galatians 6:8

Goals for Thursday:

Physical: _____
_____
_____

Mental: _____
_____
_____

Spiritual: _____
_____
_____

What are 5 things I accomplished in the last year? _____
_____
_____
_____
_____
_____
_____

What am I thankful for today? _____
_____
_____

One nice thing I've done for myself today... _____
_____
_____

Day: Thursday

		Carbs	Calories
Meal 1	2 eggs	0	150
	3 sausage links	0	200
	1 piece Holland Rusk Dry Toast	6	30
Meal 2	2 Keebler Harvest Bakery Multigrain crackers	11	70
	2 tablespoons vegetable cream cheese	2	90
	1/2 cup cubed watermelon	6	25
Meal 3	6 ounces chicken breast, broiled	0	186
	1 cup steamed broccoli	FREE	FREE
	1 tablespoon butter	0	102
Meal 4	Curves shake with 8 oz. skim milk	FREE	FREE
Meal 5	1 serving Beef and Vegetable Stew (recipe page 66)	8	256
	Free Foods Salad		
	Salad Dressing (your choice)		
Meal 6	1 ounce dry roasted peanuts	5	160
	2 ounces Cheddar cheese	0	220
	1 peach	9	37

Water: 🥛🥛🥛🥛🥛🥛🥛🥛

Vitamins: 💊💊💊

Totals for Day

Today's Exercise:

Curves Workout ♡

or

Aerobic ♡

_____

_____

Strength Training ♡

_____

_____

Stretching ♡

_____

_____

...a time to be born and a time to die, a time to plant and a time to uproot, a time to kill and a time to heal, a time to tear down and a time to build...

Ecclesiastes 3:2-3

Goals for Friday:

Physical: _____

_____

_____

Mental: _____

_____

_____

Spiritual: _____

_____

_____

Am I most comfortable when everything around me stays exactly the same? _____

_____

_____

_____

_____

_____

_____

What am I thankful for today? _____

_____

_____

One nice thing I've done for myself today... _____

_____

_____

_____

Day: Friday

		Carbs	Calories
Meal 1	2 eggs	0	150
	2 ounces lean ham	0	67
	1 slice whole wheat bread	12	70
	1/2 tablespoon butter	0	51
Meal 2	Curves shake with 8 oz. skim milk	FREE	FREE
Meal 3	2 Turkey-Lettuce Wraps (recipe page 59)	4	152
	1/2 cup strawberries	6	23
Meal 4	2 ounces Cheddar cheese	0	220
	2 Rye Krisp crackers	11	60
Meal 5	8 ounces salmon, broiled	0	414
	1 cup steamed asparagus	FREE	FREE
	1/2 tablespoon butter	0	51
	Free Foods Salad		
	Salad Dressing (your choice)		
Meal 6	1/2 cup 1% fat cottage cheese	5	80
	1/2 cup cubed cantaloupe	6	25
	1 ounce roasted and salted cashews	7	170

Water: 🥛🥛🥛🥛🥛🥛🥛🥛

Vitamins: ⊖ ⊖ ⊖

Totals for Day

TIP:
Try melting your cheese on Rye-Krisp crackers. You can do it quickly in the microwave. Many cheeses taste quite different when melted.

PHASE II - 4

161

"Inaction saps the vigor of the mind."

—Leonardo da Vinci

Goals for Saturday:

Physical: _____

_____

Mental: _____

_____

Spiritual: _____

_____

_____

How many hours per week do I watch TV? Am I really
enjoying it or am I doing it because of habit? _____

_____

_____

_____

_____

_____

_____

_____

What am I thankful for today? _____

_____

_____

One nice thing I've done for myself today... _____

_____

_____

_____

Day: Saturday

		Carbs	Calories
Meal 1	1 slice whole wheat bread	12	70
	1 ounce Havarti cheese	0	120
	3 sausage links	0	200
Meal 2	Curves shake with 8 oz. skim milk	FREE	FREE
Meal 3	6 ounces 93% lean ground beef, broiled	0	240
	1 ounce Cheddar cheese	0	110
	$1/2$ cup refried beans	25	120
	2 tablespoons salsa	2	10
Meal 4	8 ounces shrimp, broiled	0	240
	1 serving Spicy Zucchini Boats (page 58)	2	195
Meal 5	Free Foods Salad		
	Salad Dressing (your choice)		
Meal 6	1 ounce dry roasted peanuts	5	160
	1 plum	9	36

Water: 🥛🥛🥛🥛🥛🥛🥛🥛

Vitamins: ⬭ ⬭ ⬭

Totals for Day

Today's Exercise:

Curves Workout ♡

or

Aerobic ♡

_____

_____

Strength Training ♡

_____

_____

Stretching ♡

_____

_____

PHASE II - 4

163

A fool gives full vent to his anger, but
a wise man keeps himself under control.

Proverbs 29:11

Goals for Sunday:

Physical: _____

_____

_____

Mental: _____

_____

_____

Spiritual: _____

_____

_____

Who or what has the capacity to make me the most angry?

_____

_____

_____

_____

_____

_____

_____

What am I thankful for today? _____

_____

_____

One nice thing I've done for myself today... _____

_____

_____

_____

Day: Sunday

		Carbs	Calories
Meal 1	2 eggs	0	150
	3 sausage links	0	200
Meal 2	1/2 cup 1% fat cottage cheese	5	80
	1/2 cup cubed cantaloupe	6	25
Meal 3	4 ounces chicken breast, broiled	0	124
	1 cup snow peas	FREE	FREE
	1/2 tablespoon butter	0	51
	1 medium orange	16	65
Meal 4	2 ounces Monterey Jack cheese	0	220
	2 Rye Krisp crackers	11	60
	4 ounce glass of rosé wine	6	100
Meal 5	8 ounces orange roughy sautéed in:	0	216
	1 tablespoon olive oil	0	120
	1 cup spinach	FREE	FREE
	Free Foods Salad		
	Salad Dressing (your choice)		
	1 serving Frozen Chocolate Mousse (page 74)	9	127
Meal 6	Curves shake with 8 oz. skim milk	FREE	FREE

Water: 🥛🥛🥛🥛🥛🥛🥛🥛

Vitamins: ⬭ ⬭ ⬭

Totals for Day

PHASE II - 4

SHOPPING LIST–PHASE II, WEEK 5

Vegetables
____ $^1/_2$ cup baby carrots
____ 3 cups broccoli florets
____ 2 cups cauliflower florets
____ 1 cup green beans
____ 1 cup mushrooms, sliced
____ $^1/_2$ cup onion
____ 1 cup snow peas
____ 1 cup zucchini, sliced

Free Foods
____ enough for 6 salads

Dairy
____ 5 tablespoons butter
____ 2 cups cottage cheese, lowfat (1%), small curd
____ 6 eggs
____ $^1/_2$ gallon milk, skim
____ 1 tablespoon blue cheese
____ 5 ounces Cheddar cheese
____ 4 ounces Swiss cheese
____ 2 tablespoons vegetable cream cheese
____ 4 ounces yogurt, plain, lowfat

Fruit
____ $^1/_2$ banana
____ $^1/_2$ grapefruit
____ $^1/_4$ cup seedless grapes
____ 3 cups strawberries
____ 1 $^1/_2$ cups watermelon, cubed

Meat
____ 20 ounces chicken breast (divided)
____ 8 ounce pork chop, lean
____ 22 ounces ground beef, 93% lean (divided)
____ 6 ounce sirloin steak, well trimmed
____ 2 ounces deli roast beef
____ 4 ounces deli turkey breast
____ 5 ounces ham, lean (divided)

____ 3 breakfast sausage links
____ 8 slices bacon
____ 8 ounces light smoked sausage
____ 8 ounces salmon
____ 8 ounces shrimp

Starches
____ 4 Rye Krisp crackers
____ 2 Keebler Harvest Bakery Multigrain crackers
____ 4 slices whole wheat bread

Other
____ 2 ounces roasted and salted almonds
____ 2 ounces pistachio nuts (in shells)
____ 1 ounce dry roasted peanuts
____ 1 ounce roasted and salted cashews
____ 1 tablespoon barbeque sauce
____ 1 tablespoon mayonnaise
____ $^1/_2$ cup chocolate ice cream
____ $^1/_2$ cup refried beans
____ 2 tablespoons salsa
____ $^1/_2$ cup sauerkraut
____ 4 ounces V-8 juice
____ 4 ounces rosé wine

Recipes this week
____ Creamy Coleslaw, page 64
____ French Onion Soup, page 65
____ Frozen Chocolate Mousse, page 74
____ Jamaican Seafood Medley, page 71
____ Sherry-Mushroom Chicken, page 70
____ Spicy Chili Pork Chops, page 69
____ Spicy Zucchini Boats, page 58
____ Spinach Salad, page 62
____ Tuna Salad, page 61

PHASE II
~ WEEK 5 ~

*If your weight loss drops below 1 pound per week
during Phase II, you should move to Phase III.
If you have reached your goal weight, you should move to Phase III.*

~

HIGHER PROTEIN/LOW CARBOHYDRATE

For the higher protein/low carbohydrate version, you should:

Enjoy unlimited amounts of lean meats, cheeses, eggs, seafood and poultry
(baked, broiled, or boiled—never fried).

Eat moderate to lower amounts of fat.
Limit your carbohydrate intake to 40-60 grams per day
(not counting free foods).

Eat, but don't cheat!

CALORIE-RESTRICTED

For the calorie-restricted version, you should:

Eat no more than 1600 calories per day
(not counting free foods).

Consume 40% of those calories in the form of protein foods.

Consume no more than 60 grams of carbohydrates per day
(not counting free foods).

~

HINT: You are not required to eat the meals in the order they are listed.
Feel free to adjust them to your lifestyle and schedule.

~
Weekly Lesson #6
~

PERMANENT RESULTS

List 3 things that are different about you since starting this 6 week challenge:

1. _____
2. _____
3. _____

List 5 foods you have truly enjoyed eating during the last 5 weeks on the plan:

1. _____
2. _____
3. _____
4. _____
5. _____

List 3 things that will be difficult about Phase III:

1. _____
2. _____
3. _____

Even if you have only lost 5 pounds over the last 5 weeks, you want to maintain that weight loss. If you have reached your goal weight, you certainly don't want to gain the weight back. Thankfully, the Curves Weight Loss Method gives us a way to eat normally most of the time and still maintain our weight. Phase III allows us to raise our metabolism to pre-dieting levels without gaining weight back to pre-diet levels.

Be aware that following Phase III is an entirely different discipline than following Phases I and II. You must weigh yourself EVERY day, at approximately the same time of day, in approximately the same circumstances. You must be prepared to do 2 or 3 days of the Phase I plan whenever you reach your "high" weight. Be sure that you eat an adequate amount and a variety of food. You will be able to eat normally and yet maintain a healthy weight.

LOOKING BACK

Think back to when you began this 6 week challenge. You have made gains in many areas of your life. You may have attained your goal weight and body fat percentage, or you may have more to accomplish. In either case, you are to be congratulated for your courage and perseverance. You have voluntarily denied yourself the short term pleasure of eating whatever you want whenever you want. You have willingly taken the time to exercise and to plan your eating. You have become comfortable with being a little bit uncomfortable.

Now you know how to follow the Curves Weight Loss Method and allow yourself to achieve Permanent Results Without Permanent Dieting. The rest is up to you. You are armed with experience and knowledge, but you will still have to choose correctly every day.

You can do it!

Name 3 things about this plan that at first seemed difficult but now seem easy:

1._____
2._____
3._____

Name 2 things about this plan that never did get to be easy:

1._____
2._____

List 6 reasons to maintain your weight loss:

1._____
2._____
3._____
4._____
5._____
6._____

"The poor man is not he who is without a cent,
but he who is without a dream."

—Harry Kemp

Goals for Monday:

Physical: _____

_____

_____

Mental: _____

_____

_____

Spiritual: _____

_____

_____

What are 10 things I want to do before I die?_____

_____

_____

_____

_____

_____

_____

_____

_____

_____

_____

What am I thankful for today? _____

_____

_____

One nice thing I've done for myself today... _____

_____

Day: Monday

		Carbs	Calories
Meal 1	4 ounces deli turkey breast	4	120
	1 ounce Swiss cheese	0	110
	1 slice whole wheat bread	12	70
	1 tablespoon mayonnaise	0	100
Meal 2	½ cup 1% fat cottage cheese	5	80
	½ cup baby carrots	5	24
Meal 3	6 ounces 93% lean ground beef, broiled	0	240
	1 serving French Onion Soup (recipe page 65)	3	145
Meal 4	⅔ cup tuna salad (recipe page 61)	3	258
	2 Rye Krisp crackers	11	60
Meal 5	1 serving Spicy Chili Pork Chops (recipe page 69)	4	219
	1 cup steamed broccoli	FREE	FREE
	1 tablespoon butter	0	102
	Free Foods Salad		
	Salad Dressing (your choice)		
Meal 6	Curves shake with 8 oz. skim milk	FREE	FREE

Water: 🥛🥛🥛🥛🥛🥛🥛
Vitamins: ⬭ ⬭ ⬭

Totals for Day

Today's Exercise:

Curves Workout ♡

or

Aerobic ♡

_____

_____

Strength Training ♡

_____

_____

Stretching ♡

_____

_____

Today you need to go to Curves to be weighed and have your body fat tested. Record your results here:

Weight _____
% Body Fat _____
Pounds of
Body Fat _____

Also record your results on the chart on page 26.

TIP:
Has eating out got you stumped?
See page 38 for some hints.

171

*So we make it our goal to please him, whether
we are at home in the body or away from it.*

2 Corinthians 5:9

Goals for Tuesday:

Physical: _____

_____

_____

Mental: _____

_____

_____

Spiritual: _____

_____

_____

What are my goals in life? For the next year? 5 years?
20 years? _____

_____

_____

_____

_____

_____

_____

_____

What am I thankful for today? _____

_____

_____

One nice thing I've done for myself today... _____

_____

_____

_____

Day: Tuesday

			Carbs	Calories
Meal 1	2 eggs		0	150
	2 ounces lean ham		0	67
Meal 2	$^1/_2$ cup 1% fat cottage cheese		5	80
	$^1/_2$ cup strawberries		6	23
Meal 3	6 ounces chicken breast, broiled		0	186
	1 serving Spinach Salad (recipe page 62)			
	with 2 tablespoons Orange Vinaigrette		3	101
	1 slice whole wheat bread		12	70
	$^1/_2$ tablespoon butter		0	51
Meal 4	Curves shake with 8 oz. skim milk		FREE	FREE
Meal 5	1 serving Jamaican Seafood Medley (recipe page 71)		6	283
	1 cup zucchini, sauteed in:		FREE	FREE
	1 tablespoon olive oil		0	120
	1 serving Frozen Chocolate Mousse (recipe page 74)		9	127
Meal 6	1 ounce Cheddar cheese		0	110
	$^1/_4$ cup seedless grapes		7	29
	1 ounce roasted and salted almonds		4	180

Water: 🥛🥛🥛🥛🥛🥛🥛

Vitamins: ⬭ ⬭ ⬭

Totals for Day

Today's Exercise:

Curves Workout ♡

or

Aerobic ♡

_____

_____

Strength Training ♡

_____

_____

Stretching ♡

_____

_____

*Are you so foolish? After beginning with
the Spirit, are you now trying to attain your
goal by human effort?*

Galatians 3:3

Goals for Wednesday:

Physical: _____
_____
_____

Mental: _____
_____
_____

Spiritual: _____
_____
_____

Look back at the goals I set for myself on page 76. How did
I do? How realistic were my goals? _____
_____
_____
_____
_____
_____
_____

What am I thankful for today? _____
_____
_____

One nice thing I've done for myself today... _____
_____
_____
_____

Day: Wednesday

		Carbs	Calories
Meal 1	4 ounces plain yogurt	9	75
	1 cup strawberries	12	46
Meal 2	Curves shake with 8 oz. skim milk	FREE	FREE
Meal 3	8 ounces lean ground beef, broiled	0	320
	2 ounces Cheddar cheese	0	220
	1/2 cup refried beans	25	120
	2 tablespoon salsa	2	10
Meal 4	1 serving Spicy Zucchini Boats (recipe page 58)	2	195
Meal 5	8 ounce pork chop, broiled	0	300
	1 cup steamed cauliflower	FREE	FREE
	1/2 tablespoon butter	0	51
	Free Foods Salad		
	Salad Dressing (your choice)		
Meal 6	2 ounces deli roast beef	2	60
	1 ounce Swiss cheese	0	110

Water: ☐ ☐ ☐ ☐ ☐ ☐ ☐ ☐
Vitamins: ☐ ☐ ☐

Totals for Day

Today's Exercise:

Curves Workout ♡

or

Aerobic ♡

_____

_____

Strength Training ♡

_____

_____

Stretching ♡

_____

_____

TIP:
Even if you consider yourself a pro at estimating food portions, it is smart to actually measure them whenever possible.

"There are only two things that prevent you from accomplishing your goals—fear and self doubt. When you learn to trust yourself and ask for help, the world gets a whole lot easier."

—Wyatt Webb

Goals for Thursday:

Physical: _____

_____

_____

Mental: _____

_____

_____

Spiritual: _____

_____

_____

What is one thing I can do in five minutes to make today simpler? (i.e. return phone calls, clean off desk, pay some bills, file papers) _____

_____

_____

_____

_____

_____

What am I thankful for today? _____

_____

_____

One nice thing I've done for myself today... _____

_____

Day: <u>Thursday</u>

		Carbs	Calories
Meal 1	1 egg	0	75
	4 slices bacon	0	120
	4 ounces V-8 juice	5	23
	$\frac{1}{2}$ banana	13	53
Meal 2	2 Keebler Harvest Bakery Multigrain crackers	11	70
	2 tablespoons vegetable cream cheese	2	90
	1 cup cubed watermelon	12	50
Meal 3	8 ounces chicken breast, broiled	0	248
	1 tablespoon blue cheese (melted on chicken)	0	30
	1 cup steamed broccoli	FREE	FREE
	$\frac{1}{2}$ tablespoon butter	0	51
Meal 4	Curves shake with 8 oz. skim milk	FREE	FREE
Meal 5	6 ounces sirloin steak, broiled	0	323
	Free Foods Salad		
	Salad Dressing (your choice)		
Meal 6	1 ounce roasted and salted almonds	4	180
	1 ounce Cheddar cheese	0	110
	4 ounce glass of rosé wine	6	100

Water: 🥛🥛🥛🥛🥛🥛🥛🥛

Vitamins: ⬭ ⬭ ⬭

Totals for Day

Today's Exercise:

Curves Workout ♡

or

Aerobic ♡

_____

_____

Strength Training ♡

_____

_____

Stretching ♡

_____

_____

"The greater part of our happiness or misery depends on our dispositions, and not on our circumstances."

—Martha Washington

Goals for Friday:

Physical: _____

_____

Mental: _____

_____

Spiritual: _____

_____

_____

What 3 things do I like about myself? _____

_____

_____

_____

_____

_____

_____

What am I thankful for today? _____

_____

_____

One nice thing I've done for myself today... _____

_____

_____

_____

_____

Day: Friday

		Carbs	Calories
Meal 1	1 egg	0	75
	3 ounces ham, lean	0	100
Meal 2	Curves shake with 8 oz. skim milk	FREE	FREE
Meal 3	8 ounces lean ground beef, broiled	0	320
	1 tablespoon barbeque sauce	6	25
	1 serving Creamy Coleslaw (recipe page 64)	3	78
Meal 4	1 ounce Swiss cheese	0	110
	2 Rye Krisp crackers	11	60
	2 ounces pistachio nuts (in shells)	7	170
Meal 5	8 ounces shrimp sautéed in:	0	240
	1 tablespoon olive oil	0	120
	1 cup green beans	8	40
	1/2 tablespoon butter	0	51
	Free Foods Salad		
	Salad Dressing (your choice)		
Meal 6	1/2 cup 1% fat cottage cheese	5	80
	1 cup strawberries	12	46

Water: ⬚ ⬚ ⬚ ⬚ ⬚ ⬚ ⬚ ⬚

Vitamins: ⬚ ⬚ ⬚

Totals for Day

Today's Exercise:

Curves Workout ♡

or

Aerobic ♡

_____

_____

Strength Training ♡

_____

_____

Stretching ♡

_____

_____

PHASE II - 5

TIP:
You need to reward yourself for making it to this point. How about a facial or a massage or a manicure?

But I have prayed for you,....that your faith may not fail. And when you have turned back, strengthen your brothers.

Luke 22:32

Goals for Saturday:

Physical: _____

_____

Mental: _____

_____

Spiritual: _____

_____

Name the 3 most difficult challenges of this diet. What can I do to improve in these areas? _____

_____

_____

_____

_____

_____

What am I thankful for today? _____

_____

_____

One nice thing I've done for myself today... _____

_____

_____

_____

Day: Saturday

		Carbs	Calories
Meal 1	1 slice whole wheat bread	12	70
	1 ounce Cheddar cheese	0	110
	3 sausage links	0	200
	1/2 grapefruit	12	46
Meal 2	Curves shake with 8 oz. skim milk	FREE	FREE
Meal 3	Free Foods Salad		
	Salad Dressing (your choice)		
Meal 4	6 ounces chicken breast, broiled	0	186
	1 cup snow peas	FREE	FREE
	1/2 tablespoon butter	0	51
Meal 5	8 ounces broiled salmon	0	414
	Stir fry of:		
	1 tablespoon olive oil	0	120
	1/2 cup onion	FREE	FREE
	1 cup mushrooms	FREE	FREE
	1 cup broccoli	FREE	FREE
Meal 6	1/2 cup chocolate ice cream	19	160
	1/2 cup strawberries	6	23
	1 ounce dry roasted peanuts	5	160

Water: ▯ ▯ ▯ ▯ ▯ ▯ ▯ ▯

Vitamins: ▭ ▭ ▭

Totals for Day

PHASE II - 5

Today's Exercise:

Curves Workout ♡

or

Aerobic ♡

_____

_____

Strength Training ♡

_____

_____

Stretching ♡

_____

_____

If you are still losing 1 to 2 pounds per week, you should continue doing Phase II. When you reach your goal weight or a plateau, go to Phase III (page 185)

"Strength is the capacity to break a chocolate bar
into four pieces with your bare hands—
and then eat just one of the pieces."

—Judith Viorst

Goals for Sunday:

Physical: _____
_____
_____

Mental: _____
_____
_____

Spiritual: _____
_____
_____

Name 3 positive behavioral changes I have made during this
diet. _____
_____
_____
_____
_____
_____
_____

What am I thankful for today? _____
_____
_____

One nice thing I've done for myself today... _____
_____
_____
_____

Day: Sunday

		Carbs	Calories
Meal 1	2 eggs	0	150
	4 slices bacon	0	120
	1 slice whole wheat bread	12	70
	1/2 tablespoon butter	0	51
Meal 2	1/2 cup 1% fat cottage cheese	5	80
	1/2 cup cubed watermelon	6	25
Meal 3	8 ounces light smoked sausage	16	440
	1/2 cup sauerkraut	FREE	FREE
	1 cup steamed cauliflower	FREE	FREE
	1/2 tablespoon butter	0	51
Meal 4	1 ounce Swiss cheese	0	110
	1 ounce roasted and salted cashews	7	170
Meal 5	1 serving Sherry-Mushroom Chicken (recipe page 70)	3	288
	Free Foods Salad		
	Salad Dressing (your choice)		
Meal 6	Curves shake with 8 oz. skim milk	FREE	FREE

Water: ☐ ☐ ☐ ☐ ☐ ☐ ☐
Vitamins: ☐ ☐ ☐

Totals for Day

Today's Exercise:

Curves Workout ♡

or

Aerobic ♡

_____

_____

Strength Training ♡

_____

_____

Stretching ♡

_____

_____

Tomorrow you need to go to Curves to be weighed, measured and have your body fat tested. Record your results here:

Weight_____

% Body Fat _____

Pounds of Body Fat _____

Record your results on the chart on page 26. You also need to have measurements taken and recorded in the chart on page 25 (Week 6 Measurements)

"The longer I live, the more I realize
the impact of attitude on life.
Attitude, to me, is more important than
education, than money, than circumstances,
than failures, than successes, than appearance,
giftedness or skill. It will make or break
a company, church or home.
The remarkable thing is that we have
a choice every day regarding the attitude
we will embrace for that day.
We cannot change our past.
We cannot change the fact that
people will act in a certain way.
We cannot change the inevitable.
The only thing we can do is play on the one
string we have, and that is our attitude.
I am convinced that life is
10% of what happens to me
and 90% how I react to it.
And so it is with you.
We are in charge of our attitudes."

–Charles Swindoll

PHASE III

*If you have more weight to lose and you are still losing
1 to 2 pounds per week, you may stay on Phase II until you
either reach your goal or you hit a plateau.*

~

You should begin Phase III if:

* You have reached your goal

* You have hit a plateau

* You are ready to take a break from dieting

~

Phase III is not really a diet, it is mostly eating.
The objective is to raise your metabolism back to pre-diet levels
without regaining the weight you lost.

The objective of Phase III is to raise metabolism back up to the level it was before you began this diet. Phase III is not really a diet; in fact, it is mostly eating. Eating is what stops the production of starvation hormones and raises metabolism.

Because your metabolic rate has decreased due to dieting, you will gain weight from eating more calories than you are burning. The first couple of pounds that you immediately gain after going off a diet are water weight. Because you no longer need to access stored energy (body fat), your body will rehydrate. The key is to not gain more weight than you can lose in a 72-hour period (3 days), because that's how long it takes for your body to begin producing starvation hormones. You must also continue to exercise at least 3 days per week to keep your metabolism high and to encourage your body to preserve its muscle mass.

PHASE III MAINTENANCE CHART EXAMPLE

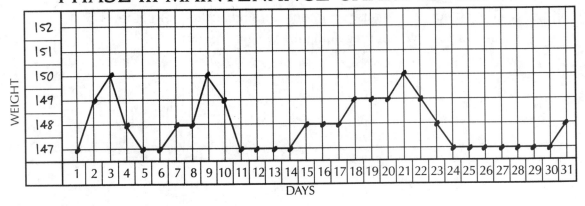

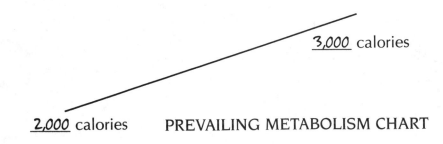

3,000 calories

2,000 calories   PREVAILING METABOLISM CHART

SUCCESS!

You have reached your goal weight and want to maintain it. Establish a low weight (your current weight) and a high weight (3-5 pounds over that). Now you must begin eating normally (2000-3000 calories per day) and you must weigh yourself every day. You will probably gain 1-2 pounds in the first day or two.

When the scale registers at the high weight, you will need to do the Phase I diet for 2-3 days, until you are back at the low weight. The 3-5 pounds you will gain probably consist of 2-3 pounds of water and 1 pound of body fat. The Phase I diet will cause you to dehydrate and burn off the body fat that you gained. Because you only do the Phase I diet for 2-3 days, you won't restimulate the production of starvation hormones. You must be sure to eat an adequate amount of food for your body size and activity level; this is the only way to raise your metabolism. Most importantly, you must never gain more weight than you can lose in 2-3 days.

Your goal is to be able to eat normally for about 29 days a month and need to diet for 2-3 days a month. The following chart will help you monitor the Phase III process. (See page 186 for an example of how to use the chart.) Record your low weight (your current weight) and your high weight (3-5 pounds more) on the left side, going up in pounds. The bottom of the chart marks off days. Start with Day 1 and make a dot at your weight. Move along the chart, following the Phase III plan by dieting when you must and eating normally otherwise. Notice that over a period of time, it will take longer and longer to gain that 3-5 pounds, so you will have more days of eating normally. You will know your prevailing metabolism by the amount of food that you can eat without gaining weight.

PHASE III MAINTENANCE CHART

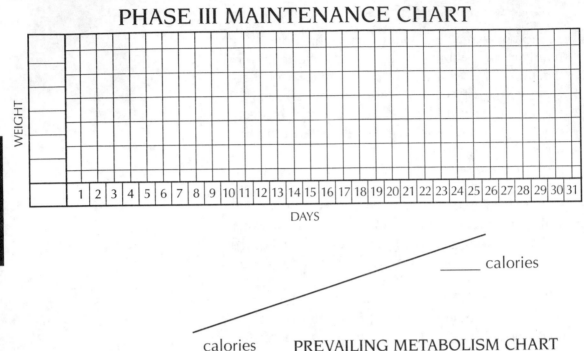

WEIGHT

| | 1 | 2 | 3 | 4 | 5 | 6 | 7 | 8 | 9 | 10 | 11 | 12 | 13 | 14 | 15 | 16 | 17 | 18 | 19 | 20 | 21 | 22 | 23 | 24 | 25 | 26 | 27 | 28 | 29 | 30 | 31 |

DAYS

_____ calories

_____ calories   PREVAILING METABOLISM CHART

MORE TO GO

You have been losing weight, but have reached a plateau and just can't seem to lose any more weight, even though you are following the Phase II plan faithfully. There is no reason to continue to diet; it is time to raise your metabolism. You need to enjoy Phase III for a month or two. This will be a time to eat healthfully and abundantly. You will raise your metabolism back to its pre-dieting level without regaining the weight you have lost. When your metabolism is sufficiently high, you should begin dieting again, starting with 1 or 2 weeks on Phase I and then moving on to Phase II.

Your metabolism is sufficiently high when you can eat 2,000-3,000 calories a day and not gain weight. It may be necessary for you to cycle through the phases several times before reaching your goal weight.

Simply follow the Phase III method previously

described. In a month or two of mostly eating, you will have stabilized at this new weight. Your metabolism should be sufficiently high to allow you to begin losing weight again.

LOW METABOLISM

If you have been yo-yo dieting or have been dieting perpetually, you may have sabotaged your metabolism. You should disregard Phases I and II and begin with Phase III in order to raise metabolism. The process is the same. Your current weight will be your low or ideal weight and you should select a high weight that is a few pounds higher. Begin to eat at a caloric level that is high enough to raise your metabolism. Never gain more than a few pounds, then lose them by using the Phase I diet for two or three days. As your prevailing metabolism is raised, you should be able to eat normally for longer periods of time, before you reach your high weight and must diet again.

When your metabolism is sufficiently high to start losing weight you may follow the normal program, beginning with Phase I.

CONGRATULATIONS

I hope you have enjoyed great success with this program. There are many ways to measure your success other than just the scale. Your clothes fit better. People are noticing that you look different. You have more energy and you feel better about yourself. Even if you are not at your ultimate goal, you have come a long way. The best part is that you need never regain any of the weight that you lost. You protected your lean tissue and have raised metabolism back to pre-diet levels.

You have set yourself up for long-term success with your health, nutrition and weight-loss goals. Enjoy it!

God Bless,

Gary Heavin,
Founder & C.E.O.
Curves International, Inc.

Aerobics (Cardio)   10
Attitude quote   184
Basic Cooking Terms   35
Basic Kitchen Tools   34
Basic Spices   36
Beef & Vegetable Stew (Recipe)   66
Beef Tenderloin with
    Blue Cheese (Recipe)   67
Calorie Sensitivity Test   29
Carbohydrate Intolerance Test   28
Carbohydrate Intolerance,
    Symptoms of   28
Carbohydrates, Explanation   14
Cardio (Aerobics)   10
Checklist, Ready to Diet   75
Cheese Chart   54
Chicken, Sherry-Mushroom (Recipe)   70
Chocolate Mousse, Frozen (Recipe)   74
Chronic Diseases   17
Coleslaw, Creamy (Recipe)   64
Congratulations   190
Cooking Terms, Basic   35
Creamy Coleslaw (Recipe)   64
Curves Complete Supplement   22
Curves Essential Supplement   23
Curves Herbal FEM Supplement   23
Curves Integrated Supplement   23
Curves PMS Formula Supplement   23
Curves Shake   23
Curves Shake Variations   43
Curves Workout   9
Dairy Products Chart   53
Dieting On The Go   37
Diets Don't Work (Weekly Lesson)   96
Don't Quit (Weekly Lesson)   115
Easy Frittata Recipe   68
Eating Out Tips   38
Embracing Change (Weekly Lesson)   78
Equivalent Measurements   34
Estimating Portions   41
Exercise Chart   27
Exercise Helps (Weekly Lesson)   114
Fats Explanation   14
Fats Chart   51
Feeding Your Family   37
Fiber   40
Food Charts:
    Cheese   54
    Dairy Products   53
    Fats   51
    Fruits   49
    Grains & Starches   52
    Miscellaneous Foods   52

    My Favorites   55
    Nuts   51
    Protein   50
    Vegetables   48
Food Diary Example   45
Food Diary, How To Use   44
Food Diary Icons, Guide to   44
Food Directory, Personal   47
Free Foods List   31
Free Foods Salad   32
French Onion Soup (Recipe)   65
Frittata, Easy (Recipe)   68
Frozen Chocolate Mousse (Recipe)   74
Fruits Chart   49
Goals Weekly Lesson   79
Grains & Starches Chart   52
Greek Salad Recipe   63
Guide to Food Diary Icons   44
Habits (Weekly Lesson)   133
How to Cook Meat and Fish   36
How to Read A Nutrition Label   42
How To Use the Food Diary Page   44
Insulin   14
Italian Stuffed Mushrooms (Recipe)   60
Jamaican Seafood Medley (Recipe)   71
Kitchen Tools, Basic   34
Lettuce Wraps, Turkey (Recipe)   59
Looking Back (Weekly Lesson)   169
Low Metabolism   189
Measurement Charts   25
Measurement Equivalents   34
Meat and Fish, How to Cook   36
Metabolism, Low   189
Minerals   57
Miscellaneous Foods Chart   52
More To Go   188
Mushrooms, Italian Stuffed (Recipe)   60
My Favorites Chart   55
Needs (Weekly Lesson)   150
Nutrition Label, How to Read   42
Nutritional Supplementation   17
Nuts Chart   51
Onion Soup, French (Recipe)   65
Orange Vinaigrette Dressing (Recipe)   62
Pantry Essentials   34
Parmesan-Vegetable Stir-Fry (Recipe)   73
Permanent Results (Weekly Lesson)   168
Personal Food Directory   47
Phase I Diet   77
Phase I Explanation   30
Phase I Summary   15
Phase I Shopping List   76
Phase I - Week 2 Diet   95

INDEX

INDEX

Phase II Explanation 15
Phase II - Week 1 Diet 95
Phase II - Week 1 Shopping List 94
Phase II - Week 2 Diet 113
Phase II - Week 2 Shopping List 112
Phase II - Week 3 Diet 131
Phase II - Week 3 Shopping List 130
Phase II - Week 4 Diet 149
Phase II - Week 4 Shopping List 148
Phase II - Week 5 Diet 167
Phase II - Week 5 Shopping List 166
Phase III Explanation 16
Phase III Maintenance Chart 188
Plateau, Reaching A 188
Pork Chops, Spicy Chili (Recipe) 69
Portions, Estimating 41
Prevailing Metabolism Chart 188
Protein Chart 50
Proteins, Explanation 14
Reach Your Goal 187
Reaching A Plateau 188
Ready to Diet Checklist 75
Recipes: Beef & Vegetable Stew 66
    Beef Tenderloin with Blue Cheese 67
    Creamy Coleslaw 64
    Easy Frittata 68
    French Onion Soup 65
    Frozen Chocolate Mousse 74
    Greek Salad 63
    Italian Stuffed Mushrooms 60
    Jamaican Seafood Medley 71
    Orange Vinaigrette Dressing 62
    Parmesan-Vegetable Stir-Fry 73
    Sherry-Mushroom Chicken 70
    Spicy Chili Pork Chops 69
    Spicy Zucchini Boats 58
    Spinach Salad 62
    Tofu Stir-Fry 72
    Tuna Salad 61
    Turkey-Lettuce Wraps 59
Resources Directory 24
Salad Dressings 33
Seafood Medley, Jamaican (Recipe) 71
Self-Labels & Self-Talk (Weekly Lesson) 132
Shake Variations 43
Sherry-Mushroom Chicken (Recipe) 70
Shopping Lists:
    Phase I 76
    Phase II - Week 1 94
    Phase II - Week 2 112
    Phase II - Week 3 130
    Phase II - Week 4 148
    Phase II - Week 5 166

Soup, French Onion (Recipe) 65
Spices, Basic 36
Spicy Chili Pork Chops (Recipe) 69
Spicy Zucchini Boats (Recipe) 58
Spinach Salad with
    Orange Vinaigrette (Recipe) 62
Starches & Grains Chart 52
Starvation Hormones 15
Stew, Beef & Vegetable (Recipe) 66
Stir-Fry, Parmesan-Vegetable (Recipe) 73
Stir-Fry, Tofu (Recipe) 72
Strength Training 11
Stretching 12
Substitutions 46
Success 187
Supplementation, Nutritional 22
Symptoms of Carbohydrate Intolerance 28
Table of Contents 3
Test 1 28
Test II 29
Test III 29
Test Results 30
The Challenge (Weekly Lesson) 97
Tips for Eating Out 38
Tofu Stir-Fry (Recipe) 72
Tuna Salad (Recipe) 61
Turkey-Lettuce Wraps (Recipe) 59
Vegetable Stir-Fry, Parmesan (Recipe) 73
Vegetables Chart 48
Vitamins 56
Wants (Weekly Lesson) 151
Water 39
Weekly Lessons:
    Diets Don't Work 96
    Don't Quit 115
    Embracing Change 78
    Exercise Helps 114
    Goals 79
    Habits 133
    Looking Back 169
    Needs 150
    Permanent Results 168
    Self-Labels & Self-Talk 132
    The Challenge 97
    Wants 151
Weight Loss Chart 26
Zucchini Boats, Spicy (Recipe) 58